MW00442704

# NATUROPATHIC
# First Aid

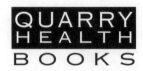

**QUARRY HEALTH BOOKS**

*Fundamentals of Naturopathic Medicine*
by Fraser Smith, ND

*The Botanical Pharmacy: The Pharmacology of Common Herbs*
by Heather Boon, BScPhm, PhD and Michael Smith, MRPharmsS, ND

*A Call to Women: A Naturopathic Guide to Preventing Breast Cancer*
by Sat Dharam Kaur, ND

*Vitamin C & Cancer*
by Abram Hoffer, MD, PhD, FRCP (C) and Linus Pauling, PhD

*Vitamin B-3 & Schizophrenia*
by Abram Hoffer, MD, PhD, FRCP (C)

*Hoffer's Laws of Natural Nutrition*
by Abram Hoffer, MD, PhD, FRCP (C)

*Dr Hoffer's ABC of Natural Nutrition for Children*
by Abram Hoffer, MD, PhD, FRCP (C)

*Masks of Madness: Science of Healing*
by Abram Hoffer, MD, PhD, FRCP (C)
(Introduction by Margot Kidder)

*Dr Max Gerson: Healing the Hopeless*
by Howard Straus

# Naturopathic First Aid

## A GUIDE

*to*

## TREATING MINOR FIRST AID CONDITIONS

*with*

## NATURAL MEDICINES

KAREN BARNES, ND

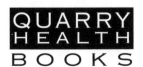

QUARRY HEALTH BOOKS

The publisher gratefully acknowledges the support of the Department of Canadian Heritage, Book Publishing Industry Development Program.

ISBN 1-55082-282-9

Cover design by Susan Hannah.

Text design and type by The Right Type.

Printed and bound in Canada by AGMV Marquis
Cap-St-Ignace, Quebec.

Published by Quarry Press Inc., P.O. Box 1061
Kingston, Ontario K7L 4Y5 Canada
www.quarrypress.com

For more information on Naturopathic First Aid, contact Karen Barnes:

www.burlingtonnaturopathic.com

or

kbarnes@burlingtonnaturopathic.com

# ❧ Contents ❧

## Dedication & Acknowledgements

I DEDICATE THIS BOOK to Steve Barnes, to my family and friends whose love and support made this possible, and especially to my daughter Julia, who after a 'boo boo' loves to slather on the calendula cream and put on a bandage. I thank Bobbi Greenberg at The Canadian College of Naturopathic Medicine for 'gently' encouraging me to write this book. I also thank Julia's care givers Steve, Chris, Tim, Iris, Elaine, and Cathy who afforded me the time to write this book. I appreciate and thank my colleagues, Dr Paul Saunders N.D., Pam Milroy N.D., Erika Ristok N.D., Nahid Ahmedzadeh N.D., and Laura Bodner N.D. for their valuable input, time and effort. Thank you also Chris Barnes and Sue MacLean for your comments.

# ✲ *Introduction* ✲

## How To Use This Book

As a naturopathic physician and a mother of two young children, I needed to put together a natural first aid kit for myself. There are so many effective natural remedies on the market that I decided to put them to the test and report the results in a book so that everyone could take advantage of the healing power of nutrients, herbs, homeopathic medicines, and acupressure techniques. It's nice to have the piece of mind that you are prepared.

This book falls into four sections. The first defines naturopathic medicine and describes the basic 'modalities' or methods of treatment and substances used, in this case, clinical nutrition, botanical medicine, essential and carrier oils, homeopathy, Bach flower remedies, and acupressure. The descriptions of these modalities can be used as a guide for choosing remedies you may want in your first aid kit and for expanding your knowledge of natural medicines.

The second section shows you how to make your own basic naturopathic first aid kit from these substances as well as customized kits for travel, sports, and outdoors activities.

The third section describes how to use your kit in treating minor conditions from bruises and burns to sprains and strains. For each ailment or injury described, a diagnostic discussion helps to distinguish serious from minor symptoms before primary and secondary treatments for minor injuries or illnesses are recommended. A fourth related section is devoted to special treatments for travel conditions. A list of companies supplying natural medicines for your first aid kit and a list of references to relevant research in naturopathic medicine complete the book.

*Naturopathic First Aid* is meant to be a complement to basic Red Cross or St John Ambulance first aid books in the treatment of minor first aid conditions. Please refer to these manuals for information on responding to such serious conditions as asphyxia and drowning, bone fractures and spinal injury, heart attacks and strokes, for example. Knowing how to bandage wounds and to use the methods of artificial respiration is essential for effective first aid treatment. And regardless of how effective naturopathic first aid may be, nothing can replace getting professional help for diagnosis and treatment of serious injuries or ailments.

Serious injury from a fall or blow, with head, chest, or abdominal trauma, with excessive bleeding or a change in behavior or consciousness,

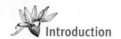 

requires immediate emergency measures. Symptoms of shock, such as paleness with sweating, cold limbs with a rapid weak pulse (where the person feels cold and clammy to the touch), and when the person feels weak and faint also require immediate emergency measures beyond primary first aid. Shock requires that the person lies down on their side with feet elevated, wrapped in a warm blanket, and monitored until emergency help arrives. If symptoms of any kind show no improvement, persist, or get worse, seek professional advice. In the case of serious emergencies, the local emergency medical service can be called and first aid can be administered while you wait for help to arrive. When in doubt, please consult a professional.

After the initial first aid measures are implemented and the crisis is dealt with, a naturopathic physician can help with selecting the proper combination of nutrition, herbs, homeopathy, acupuncture, or gentle hands-on technique that may speed the healing process further. With at least three years of university training, four years of naturopathic college and licensing examinations before opening a practice, naturopathic physicians are reliable professionals to consult. Please take advantage of their service, which is covered by most extended health insurance plans.

# What Is Naturopathic Medicine?

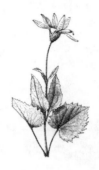

# What Is Naturopathic Medicine?

NATUROPATHIC MEDICINE IS THE USE of a variety of natural medicines to support and stimulate the body to heal itself. In addition to this principle, naturopathic medicine recognizes the individuality of each patient. Diagnostic assessment by a naturopathic physician often requires an in-depth interview and appropriate physical exam to identify the underlying cause of the disease. Treatment is individualized to the patient; those with the same condition may receive different medicines. Naturopathic doctors also practice preventative medicine by teaching their patients how to live a healthy life-style.

## Principles of Naturopathic Medicine

- First, do no harm
- Co-operate with the healing powers of nature
- Address the fundamental causes of disease
- Heal the whole person through individualized treatment
- Teach the principles of healthy living and preventative medicine

Many people with diverse conditions seek the help of a naturopathic physician. Often, patients consulting a naturopathic physician have chronic problems, such as recurrent ear infections, auto-immune disease, premenstrual syndrome (PMS), or arthritis. Naturopathic medicine can also be used in the treatment of acute conditions, such as colds and flu, as well as some minor first aid conditions by supporting and stimulating the body to heal itself naturally, without the use of drugs or surgery. Nevertheless, naturopathic medicine does not replace these other forms of health care; rather, it complements them. This naturopathic first aid book, for example, complements Red Cross or St John Ambulance approaches to minor conditions.

Training for naturopathic medicine is extensive. A three-year degree of pre-med study at university is followed by a four-year full-time program at a naturopathic college. In most provinces or states, a naturopathic physician must also pass licensing exams (such as NPLX in some states and provinces in North America) before being allowed to practice.

Naturopathic medicine borrows from many ancient healing traditions. Naturopathic physicians are trained in the use of clinical nutrition, botanical or herbal medicine, homeopathic medicine, traditional Chinese medicine and acupuncture, hands-on techniques, and lifestyle counseling. After an initial assessment, which includes a physical exam, a naturopathic physician may prescribe one or a combination of these natural medicines to support the body's own healing capacity.

Clinical nutrition is the use of diet, vitamins, and minerals to prevent and treat diseases. Nutrition is the foundation of good health since nutrients are the building blocks of the body. Vitamins and minerals are co-factors for many enzyme systems in the body, including detoxification and repair of tissue. For example, vitamin A, vitamin C, vitamin E, and zinc are all necessary for tissue repair from wounds and burns. After a wound or burn, increasing these vitamins and minerals can greatly enhance the body's ability to heal. Clinical nutrition, based on scientific studies, also takes into account the form of the vitamin or mineral that will give the best absorption and assimilation into the body.

There are three ways to use nutrition in naturopathic medicine: to meet the recommended daily allowance (RDA), to achieve an optimal daily allowance (ODA), or to treat disease with therapeutic doses (TD). Many people today, although they may be getting a recommended daily allowance of nutrients from their diet (a requirement set as the amount of vitamins and minerals needed by the average person to prevent deficiency), are not meeting their optimal daily allowance of nutrients. Optimizing nutrition allows the body to maintain health, overcome illness more effectively, and even prevent disease. This dose may not be available through diet alone, thus requiring supplementation. Vitamins can also be used in therapeutic doses (much higher than the RDA or ODA doses) for a short period of time under the supervision of a naturopathic physician to aid in the treatment of many conditions.

Herbal or botanical medicine has been used all over the world for thousands of years and still is the primary medicine for 80 percent of the world's population. Before the advent of modern drugs, people used plants indigenous to their area to treat a range of conditions. Echinacea spp. (purple coneflower), for example, has been used in the treatment of colds and flu for centuries. We now know that echinacea increases white blood cell count as one of its mechanisms of action.

Another form of botanical medicine is the use of 'essential' and 'carrier' oils. Essential oils are volatile oils of plants that escape into the air and can be used by the plants themselves to ward off predators or attract pollinating insects. When derived from a plant, essential oils are very concentrated and are generally only applied topically on the skin and not taken internally. Lavender oil, for example, is used to calm the nervous system, and can be either massaged onto the temples to treat a headache, or dropped onto a cloth with a dropper and put inside a pillowcase to aid falling asleep. External application of lavender essential oil is also useful to promote wound healing for minor burns and cuts. Tea tree essential oil has a history of use as an antibacterial and antifungal when applied topically to minor cuts and local fungal infections. Because essential oils are so potent, they often need to be diluted in a 'carrier' oil. Vegetable oils or nut oils work well as carrier oils. At home you may use corn oil, olive oil, or canola oil to dilute essential oils. To keep in a first aid kit, almond oil can be purchased in small bottles as a carrier oil.

Homeopathy — the use of minute amounts of plant, mineral, and animal substances — is relatively new, founded as a practice of medicine by physician Samuel Hahnemann in Germany during the early nineteenth century. Hahnemann believed that homeopathic medicines could be used to stimulate the body's vital force or healing capacity. Homeopathic medicine is based on the principle that 'like cures like' — the substance that produces symptoms in a healthy person can cure those same symptoms in a sick person if given in minute doses. For example, Hahnemann tested the Cinchona bark which was used to treat malaria on himself and found that the symptoms of an intermittent fever occurred when he took the herb in large doses. Thus, Cinchona bark, taken in large doses, could make a healthy person sick. After this experience, Hahnemann conducted experiments known as 'provings' on volunteers and himself to determine any changes caused by minute doses of different substances. Today, homeopathy is widely used in most European countries, India, Africa, and Australia.

The flowering parts of plants have also been used for centuries for their calming effects on emotions. A British physician, Dr Edward Bach, rediscovered in the 1920s what was previously practiced by Australian Aborigines and Native Americans, the healing power of flower essences. Bach observed that people with physical ailments also had certain associated emotions, such as anger, resentment, anxiety, and depression. Bach believed that the cause of illness is the negative thought patterns behind the feelings. He understood that treating the emotional state of the person by balancing the emotions allows for illness to resolve. These flower remedies are made from diluted essences of plants that are preserved in an alcohol-based solution. Like homeopathic remedies, Bach flower essences require a careful matching of symptoms of the flower essence with the emotions of the person. For example, the feeling of homesickness or 'living in the past' are key features indicating the need for the flower essence of Honeysuckle. "Rescue Remedy®" is a useful first aid combination of Bach flower essences for treating nervousness, trembling, anxiety, and fear.

As part of traditional Chinese medicine, acupuncture has been used in Asia for thousands of years. This diagnostic and treatment practice is based on the principle that energy or 'Qi' moves along channels through the body and that disease is caused by the blockage of energy. When acupuncture points, which arise near the skin's surface, are stimulated by tiny needles, there is a more even energy flow and a balancing of the function of the organs, cells, and tissues of the body. Acupressure, the use of pressure at these same energy points without needles, can be used at home with similar effects.

*Naturopathic First Aid* brings these natural medicines to bear upon the treatment of minor first aid conditions, first describing the injury or ailment, then distinguishing between the signs and symptoms of minor and serious injuries, before suggesting primary and secondary treatments. Our hope is that *Naturopathic First Aid* will help to ease the pain of these minor conditions and enable the body to heal.

# Vitamins & Minerals

Vitamins and minerals can be used for first aid as a support to the body's ability to heal itself. There are several key vitamins and minerals which facilitate healing, such as vitamin A, C, E, zinc, bioflavanoids, and essential fatty acids. Deficiencies of some of these nutrients have been shown to impair healing, so having recommended or optimal amounts of these nutrients may be an important element in the healing process. It is best to consult your naturopathic doctor before taking supplements, especially if you are pregnant.

Vitamin and mineral supplements are commonly available in capsule or tablet form, while bioflavinoids, such as rutin, hesperetin, hesperidin, and quercetin, are usually found together with a vitamin supplement, most commonly vitamin C. Essential fatty acids are available in black currant oil, flax seed oil, and evening primrose oil capsules or liquid.

*Note:* the doses given are for adults.

**Vitamin A**

**Form:** capsule, tablet.
**Action:** growth and repair of new tissue, antioxidant, enhances immunity.
**Indications:** burns and scalds, poison plants, scrapes, sunburn.
**Dose:** 10,000 IU, 3 times a day for 2 weeks.
**Caution:** not to be taken over 10,000 IU if pregnant or you have liver disease. Vitamin A can be toxic if taken in large doses for extended periods.

**Vitamin C (Ascorbic Acid)**

**Form:** tablet, capsule, powder.
**Action:** promotes formation of collagen and elastin in skin, antioxidant, helps to prevent bruising.
**Indications:** bruising, burns and scalds, insect bites and stings, nosebleeds, poison ivy, scrapes, sprains and strains, sunburn.
**Dose:** 500 mg, 4 times a day with food for 2–4 weeks.
**Caution:** chewable vitamin C can damage tooth enamel and lead to cavity formation. Do not exceed 4,000 mg of vitamin C if pregnant. Do not combine with aspirin as stomach irritation or ulceration may occur.
**Note:** easy bruising may signal a deficiency in vitamin C.

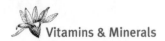 

**℞ Vitamin E**

**Form:** internally, capsules; topically, break open a capsule or apply oil from a container.
**Action:** antioxidant, facilitates tissue repair, reduces scarring, strengthens capillaries.
**Indications:** burns and scalds, scrapes, sunburn.
**Dose:** 400 IU internally. Topically apply a thin layer of oil to affected area.
**Caution:** internally, vitamin E in large doses can elevate blood pressure. Do not take large doses of vitamin E (over 1000 IU) if on blood thinners.
**Contraindication:** externally, do not use immediately on 2nd or 3rd degree burns until the top layer of skin is healing over.

**℞ Mineral Zinc**

**Form:** tablet, capsule.
**Action:** antioxidant, repair of tissue especially for collagen formation in skin and protein synthesis.
**Indications:** burns and scalds, poison ivy, scrapes, sunburn.
**Dose:** 30 mg per day for 2–4 weeks.
**Caution:** zinc supplements can cause nausea if taken in doses higher than 30 mg at one time. Do not take more than 100 mg of zinc per day.
**Note:** poor wound healing is one sign of deficiency of zinc.

**℞ Bioflavanoids (rutin, hesperetin, hesperidin, quercetin)**

**Form:** tablet, capsule (usually found together in a vitamin with vitamin C).
**Action:** reduces capillary fragility, antioxidant.
**Indications:** bruising, burns and scalds, insect bites and stings, nosebleeds, poison ivy, scrapes, sprains and strains, sunburn.
**Dose:** 1000 mg per day.
**Caution:** very high doses may cause diarrhea.

## Essential Fatty Acids
### (from black currant oil, flax seed oil, evening primrose oil)

**Form:** capsules.

**Action:** needed for repair of cells.

**Indications:** burns and scalds, poison ivy, scrapes, sunburn.

**Dose:** 1000 mg, 3 times a day with food.

**Caution:** consult your naturopathic doctor before taking if you are on anti-clotting medication (blood thinners).

**Note:** a deficiency of essential fatty acids may be a cause of poor wound healing.

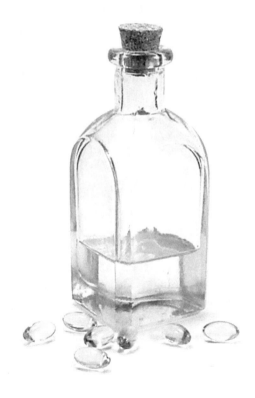

# Botanical & Herbal Remedies

Plants have been used for centuries in all cultures for their healing properties, not only for minor first aid treatment but also for more serious acute and chronic illness. Today, herbs or botanicals are available in a variety of forms besides their fresh or dried state and can be applied or ingested several ways. The following definitions provide the necessary vocabulary for discussing the medical use of herbs for first aid.

**Compress:** a cloth pad soaked in a herbal solution and applied to the skin.

**Creams:** a mixture of a herb with water and fats or oils that disperse into the skin. Creams are often used as moisturizers which penetrate and fats provide a protective layer to keep moisture in.

**Distillate:** a steam-evaporated substance in a liquid form.

**Gel:** a water-based substance made from a herb that can adhere to the skin.

**Ointment:** a mixture of a herb with only fats or oils and no water. Ointments form a separate protective layer over the skin and are good for chapped skin.

**Tincture:** an extraction of the herb using alcohol and water. Alcohol is added both to extract components of the herb and as a preservative.

## Healing Herbs for First Aid Conditions

The following list of herbs describes in detail good first aid botanicals, their properties, indications, doses, contraindications, and cautions, where applicable. The common name of each herb is given as well as the Latin or scientific name with the genus and species. You can use this section to choose the herbs you may want to have on hand in your first aid kit. For more information on the pharmacology of common herbs, *The Botanical Pharmacy*, by Heather Boon and Michael Smith, is highly recommended.

Most of these herbal remedies are available at local health food stores, though some may need to be special ordered from a herbal remedy supplier listed in the 'Naturopathic Medicine Suppliers Directory' at the back of this book or from a naturopathic doctor or other health care professional.

### Aloe gel: *Aloe vera gel*

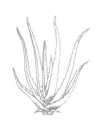

**Form:** leaf pulp, gel, or ointment.
**Topical Action:** wound healing, antifungal.
**Dose:** apply the gel or pulp of a broken aloe leaf liberally or use a store-bought gel or ointment.
**Indications:** pain relief for burns, wounds, sunburns, insect bites, fungal infections.
**Caution:** use the inside pulp and juice of the aloe plant, not the outside skin of the leaf, which has different properties.

### Arnica: *Arnica montana*

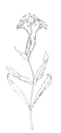

**Form:** cream, tincture, compress.
**Topical Action:** analgesic, anti-inflammatory.
**Indications:** bruises.
**Dosage:** as a cream apply to bruised area liberally; as a compress mix 1 tbsp tincture to 1 cup of water pour onto a towel and hold next to the bruised area.
**Caution:** do not use on broken skin; do not take internally.
**Note:** some people are sensitive to herbal arnica, observe for a skin rash.

### Bilberry Berries: *Vaccinium myrtillus*

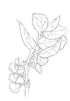

**Form:** dried berries.
**Actions:** anti-diarrheic, astringent, antibiotic, antiseptic.
**Indications:** for diarrhea such as bacterial dysentery.
**Dosage:** boil 1 tbsp berries in 1 cup of water for 10 minutes, strain and drink liquid 3–6 times a day.

### Calendula (Pot Marigold): *Calendula officinalis*

**Form:** tincture, cream, fresh leaves, flowers.
**Topical Action:** wound healing, antiseptic.
**Indications:** useful on burns and abrasions to speed tissue healing and as an antiseptic.
**Dosage:** for wound cleaning use 10 drops in 1 cup of water; as a cream, apply to area liberally.

**Contraindication:** do not use on deep wounds as calendula will heal the top layer before the bottom layers of tissue have healed, thus improperly speeding the healing process.

## ℞ Citrus Concentrates:
## Citricidal™ Liquid Concentrate (Professional Brand)

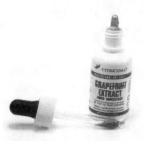

**Form:** liquid concentrate.
**Action:** antibacterial, antifungal.
**Dose:** 3–5 drops in 5–6 oz of water, in morning to prevent traveler's diarrhea, 2–3 times daily to treat diarrhea.
**Caution:** avoid contact with eyes. Do not use undiluted.
**Note:** available from a naturopathic doctor or health care professional.

## ℞ Citrus Concentrates:
## Nutribiotic™ Liquid Grapefruit Seed Extract

**Form:** liquid concentrate.
**Action:** antibacterial, antifungal.
**Dose:** 5–15 drops in 5–6 oz of water, in morning to prevent traveler's diarrhea, 2–3 times daily to treat diarrhea.
**Caution:** avoid contact with eyes. Do not use undiluted.
**Note:** available from health food stores.

## ℞ Fennel Seed: *Foeniculum vulgare*

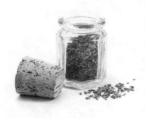

**Form:** tincture, dried seeds (tea).
**Action:** anti-spasmodic, anti-inflammatory, appetite stimulant.
**Indications:** useful for diarrhea since it removes colic and gas.
**Dosage:** 10–60 drops of tincture 3 times a day; or make a tea by pouring 1 cup of water over 1–2 tsp of crushed seeds let steep for 10 minutes.
**Contraindication:** None known.

## Ginger: *Zingiber officinalis*

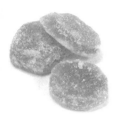

**Form:** crystallized root, thinly sliced in warm water.
**Actions:** prevents vomiting, antispasmodic, antiseptic, circulatory stimulant, promotes sweating.
**Indications:** nausea of travel sickness or morning sickness in pregnancy.
**Dose:** crystallized ginger chewed during a journey for travel sickness.
**Caution:** avoid excessive amounts of ginger with stomach ulcers, inflammation of the digestive tract, and in early pregnancy.

## Goldenseal: *Hydrastis canadensis*

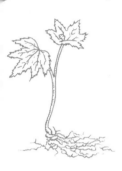

**Form:** tincture.
**Actions:** astringent, antispasmodic, antiseptic, antibiotic, hypoglycemic, healing to mucous membranes, reduces phlegm.
**Indications:** diarrhea, mucous conditions of respiratory or digestive tract. *In vitro* it has been shown to have antibiotic effects against several bacteria, protozoa, and fungi, including salmonella typhi, vibrio cholera, shigella dysenteriae, giardia lamblia.
**Dosage:** tincture 1 ml (20 drops) 3 times a day.
**Contraindication:** do not take if pregnant or lactating; avoid if you have high blood pressure; in sensitive individuals, goldenseal may cause hypoglycemia.
**Caution:** do not take for more than one week at a time. If you have glaucoma, cardiovascular disease, or diabetes, consult a naturopathic physician before using goldenseal.
**Note:** because goldenseal is antibiotic, it is important always to replace beneficial intestinal flora after its use (e.g., lactobacillus acidophilus or a combination of lactobacillus acidophilus and lactobacillus bifidus).

## ℞ Peppermint: *Mentha piperita*

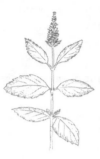

**Form:** tincture, fresh or dried leaves (tea)
**Actions:** antispasmodic, prevents vomiting, mild anesthetic antimicrobial, promotes sweating.
**Indications:** colic with gas, nausea, vomiting.
**Dose:** 1–2 ml tincture 3 times a day; or make a tea by pouring 1 cup of boiling water over 1 teaspoonful of fresh or dried leaves and steeping for 10 minutes.
**Caution:** peppermint taken over long periods may interfere with iron absorption, do not give to children under 12; do not give to babies; do not use if breast feeding as too much can reduce milk flow.
**Contraindications:** do not use if you have a hiatal hernia.

## ℞ St. John's Wort: *Hypericum perforatum*

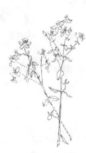

**Forms:** tincture.
**Topical Actions:** anti-inflammatory, astringent, wound healing, antimicrobial.
**Indications:** speeds the healing of wounds, bruises, and minor sunburns.
**Dosage:** 10 drops of tincture in 1 cup of water to clean a wound; Apply a gauze soaked in tincture to wounds, bruises, minor (first degree) sunburns.

## ℞ Witch Hazel: *Hamamelis virginiana*

**Form:** distillate, tincture, witch hazel water.
**Actions:** wound healing, astringent, anti-inflammatory.
**Indications:** contusions, bruising, muscle soreness, minor burns and sunburns, insect bites, hemorrhoids, varicose veins.
**Dosage:** soak a gauze pad in distilled witch hazel and apply to the bruise, muscle, sunburn, or insect bite.

# Essential & Carrier Oils

Essential oils are the volatile parts of plants or 'essences' that escape into the air giving the plant or flower its characteristic odor. These oils are very concentrated extracts made through a distillation process. These oils can be used for aromatherapy, to ward off insects, to stimulate the immune system, and topically as antifungals, antiseptics, and anti-inflammatories. General contraindications for all essential oils are, if skin irritation occurs, discontinue use; do not use internally. Some essential oils need to be diluted before being put on the skin, especially for those with sensitive skin. Carrier oils are oils which have no medicinal qualities but are used to dilute or 'carry' the essential oils. Dilution of essential oil in a carrier oil can be done by placing 2–3 drops of essential oil in one teaspoon of a carrier oil such as a vegetable oil or nut oil like almond oil, apricot kernel oil, corn oil, grape seed oil, olive oil. The following can be used on all skin types.

## Carrier Oils

**Almond Oil**
**Indications:** anti-inflammatory, emollient.
**Caution:** external use only, do not use if you have an allergy to almonds.

**Apricot Kernel Oil**
**Indications:** for sensitive dry skin, emollient.
**Caution:** external use only.

**Corn Oil**
**Indications:** emollient.

**Grape Seed Oil**
**Indications:** emollient
**Caution:** external use only.

**Olive Oil**
**Indications:** emollient.

## Essential Oils

**Citronella Oil**
**Actions:** insect deterrent.
**Indications:** helps prevent mosquito bites by providing an unpleasant odor to insects.

**Dose:** apply diluted essential oil to exposed areas.
**Dilution:** 5 drops in a 2 oz. spray bottle of water or 5 drops in 1 oz. of carrier oil.
**Application:** the spray bottle must be shaken before sprayed on the skin. Re-apply every 20 minutes, as the scent wears off.
**Caution:** keep away from face and eyes. Do not take internally.

℞ **Lavender**

**Actions:** wound healing, relieves itch and sting of insect bites, sedative, calming, antiseptic, analgesic.
**Indications:** minor burns and scalds, minor cuts and scrapes, muscle cramps, headache, insect bites, to aid falling asleep and to relax muscles.
**Dose:** for burns, a few drops of lavender oil in 1 tsp aloe vera gel for a small area, more for a larger one. Apply 2–3 drops of lavender oil in 1 tsp carrier oil for minor cuts and scrapes, massage into muscle cramps, massage onto temples and neck to relieve headache, or add to bath water to relax.
**Caution:** external use only.

℞ **Tea Tree Oil**

**Actions:** antibacterial, antifungal, antiseptic, analgesic, anti-inflammatory, wound healing.
**Indications:** minor cuts and abrasions.
**Dose:** can be used undiluted on skin. Place a few to several drops on a minor cut, scrape, or fungal patch.
**Caution:** external use only. This may sting if used undiluted on a cut or abrasion.

℞ **Vitamin E Oil**

**Form:** oil.
**Actions:** antioxidant, wound healing.
**Indications:** wound or burn healing to prevent scarring.
**Dose:** cover the affected area with a thin layer of oil.
**Contraindications:** do not use immediately on 2nd or 3rd degree burns until the top layer of skin is healing over.

# Homeopathic Remedies

Small doses of plant, animal, and mineral substances effectively stimulate the body's normal healing process. Homeopathy is based on the principle that a substance that can produce symptoms in a healthy person can cure those same symptoms in a sick person if given in minute doses. For example, a person might take homeopathic onion for hay fever symptoms like those produced in a healthy person when cutting an onion, such as watery eyes and runny nose. Like Bach flower remedies, homeopathic remedies can be given based on emotional symptoms. Arnica, for example, is often given for the emotion of shock following an injury, but can also be used as a first remedy for bruising or any trauma.

When choosing a homeopathic medicine, the symptoms of an illness must be matched to the symptoms of the medicine. For instance, the feeling of the injury, what makes it better or worse, and the emotional symptoms are all used to determine the correct remedy for that person. An example is the homeopathic remedy Rhus toxicodendron (useful for sprains and strains), when the feeling of the injury is stiffness, the pain is around the joint is achy, feels sore and bruised; when the pain is worse on first motion but better after continuous movement; when the joint feels worse from cold and damp weather; and when the emotion or overall state involves the person feeling restless with the pain. This remedy can be compared to the homeopathic remedy Bryonia, another choice for sprains and strains, when the pain is stitching, worse with the slightest motion, and the person is irritable and resentful of being fussed over.

## Composition and Potency

Homeopathic remedies are made through a series of dilutions. These medicines are prepared by diluting and percussing or banging so that the substance leaves a 'fingerprint' in the solution. Some remedies can be purchased as liquid and others are in the form of granules or pellets of milk sugar (lactose) in which the liquid has been poured over the pellets.

It is important to handle homeopathic remedies as little as possible. Homeopathic remedies can be antidoted by strong smells so it is best not to take them or store them near such things as camphor, menthol, eucalyptus and not in a first aid kit containing essential oils. They are best stored in a cool, dry place away from bright light. Homeopathic medicines have a long shelf life. These medicines will last for a lifetime.

There are several potencies (strengths or dilutions) usually recommended for first aid situations, including 12X, 30X, 6C, 12C, 30C, 200C. Dilutions of 'X' refer to a dilution series based on 1 drop of the remedy in 9 drops of water-alcohol solution; 12X means the dilution succession was done 12 times. The C or K dilutions use a ratio of 1 drop of remedy in 99 drops of solution. The number in front of the X or C indicates how many times the remedy was diluted. With each successive step, the homeopathic medicines become more potent. The 200C is a higher potency (strength) than the 12X, and as a general rule needs to be repeated less often and has a longer lasting and deeper effect than the 12X.

## Dosage

When using liquid remedies, a single dose consists of placing 1–3 drops directly under the tongue or putting the drops in a small amount of water. When using pellets, pour 1–3 pellets into the lid and empty this in the mouth so they can dissolve under the tongue. Let the medicine dissolve under the tongue and do not wash them down with a drink. While it is best to take homeopathic medicines 15 minutes away from food or drink, in a first aid situation, give the medicine as soon as possible.

In most cases, 1 dose (3 small pellets) should be used immediately. If there is improvement, do not repeat the dose unless symptoms return or if full recovery is not reached after some improvement. If the symptoms get worse immediately and then better after a few to 15 minutes for an acute injury, then you have selected the correct remedy and repetition is not necessary until symptoms worsen. Aggravation or worsening followed by improvement can occur after administering a homeopathic medicine and is an indication of correct medicine. If there is no aggravation effect, but the person feels better, then this is an indication that the remedy is working and further doses are not necessary at this time. If the person does not show improvement, then reassess the symptoms and decide if a different remedy is more appropriate.

How often a homeopathic medicine is given (repetition) depends on the potency or strength of a remedy and the severity of the injury. A remedy that is of a low potency (6X or 12X) may need to be repeated more often than a higher potency (30C or 200C). If the injury is more severe, a low potency will need to be repeated more frequently and a higher potency will probably have a better effect. For first aid situations, keep these general rules in mind and follow the guidelines recommended for each injury. If you use homeopathic medicines of a certain strength over and over again, you may need to increase the strength to get the same effect. You may wish to consult a naturopathic physician to determine if this is the case for you.

In each first aid situation, it is important to evaluate and re-evaluate the symptoms and severity of the injury. After one dose of the homeopathic medicine is given, symptoms may get better and no further doses are needed until symptoms return indicating another dose needs to be taken. Re-evaluation is also critical because after an initial dose of a homeopathic medicine, the person's symptoms may change and a different homeopathic medicine may be necessary.

## Aggravation

The term 'aggravation' in homeopathy means a brief worsening of symptoms which then resolves within a few minutes to several hours. This is a good sign that the remedy is working and no more doses should be given until a second worsening occurs after the improvement.

# Homeopathic Medicines for First Aid Conditions

This is an alphabetical list of the homeopathic medicines used in this book to treat common ailments. You can use this section to choose the remedies you may want to have on hand in your first aid kit. While some of these remedies may be available in pharmacies and health food stores, they can be ordered directly from the homeopathic remedy suppliers listed in the 'Naturopathic Medicine Suppliers Directory' at the back of this book.

### *Aconitum napellus* (**Monkshood**)

> **General use and quality:** for mental shock and fear immediately after an injury or traumatic event.
> **Mental-Emotional:** anxiety and restlessness after an injury or fright.
> **Worse:** after exposure to cold dry wind.

### Apis mellifica (Honey Bee)

**General use and quality:** insect stings where the pain is stinging and burning and there is much swelling that comes on quickly. The area feels hot to the touch. The person will not be thirsty.

**Mental-Emotional:** there may be restlessness and irritability.

**Better:** from applying cold to the area.

**Worse:** from touching or applying heat to the area.

**Note:** Apis homeopathic remedy is safe to take by those with allergies to bee stings as the homeopathic medicine is diluted. Do not take below 30C during pregnancy.

### Anacardium (Marking Nut)

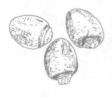

**General use and quality:** for skin rash due to poison ivy, poison oak, poison sumac with extremely itchy rash that has a yellow discharge from the blisters.

**Generally:** the person may be so itchy that they scratch until they bleed.

**Better:** the skin feels better from applying hot water.

**Worse:** the skin feels painful from scratching.

### Arnica montana (Leopard's Bane)

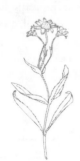

**General use and quality:** initial trauma of an injury. Bruising of the skin, head injury, blunt trauma to eye, sprains with bruising, nosebleeds from an injury or blowing the nose too hard. The part feels sore or bruised 'as if beaten'. Everything feels too hard. Jet lag.

**Mental-Emotional:** mental shock after an injury or accident. In this state, the person may deny pain or injury even after a serious injury.

**Better:** starting to move.

**Worse:** continued movement, slight pressure, heat.

### Argentum nitricum (Nitrate of Silver)

**General use and quality:** fear of flying with trembling and impulsive thoughts.

**Mental-Emotional:** fear of heights and claustrophobia, nervousness, extreme anxiety.
**Better:** fresh air.
**Worse:** warmth.

### *Arsenicum album* (Arsenious Acid)

**General use and quality:** fear of flying with restlessness and fear of death; diarrhea from food poisoning, cholera.
**General symptoms:** burning pains, thirsty for small sips frequently
**Mental-Emotional:** anxiety, nervousness, fear of death
**Better:** heat, warmth.
**Worse:** 12 p.m. to 3 a.m., cold, being alone.

### *Belladonna* (Deadly Nightshade)

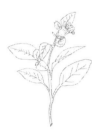

**General use and quality:** heat exhaustion or heatstroke that comes on suddenly when the person has a throbbing headache, the skin is hot and dry; sunburn where the skin feels hot and dry; a nosebleed that comes on suddenly where the blood is hot and clots easily.
**General symptoms:** the person has a red flushed face with dilated pupils.
**Mental-Emotional:** in heat exhaustion or heatstroke, the person may be delirious, have hallucinations or lose consciousness.
**Better:** warmth.
**Worse:** movement, jarring, noise, light.

### *Bryonia alba* (Wild Hops)

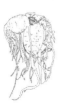

**General use and quality:** sprains and strains where the injured part is hot, red, and swollen, and the pain is of a stitching, tearing quality; heat exhaustion or heatstroke with a severe headache and possible nausea.
**Generally:** the person may feel very thirsty.
**Mental-Emotional:** the person is irritable.

**Better:** the pain is better from rest, hard pressure and applying something cold.
**Worse:** the pain is worse with the slightest motion.

### ℞ *Calendula officinalis* (Marigold)

**General use and quality:** for cuts and abrasions and slow healing wounds where the pain may be out of proportion to the injury. Infected cuts with pus.
**Better:** lying still.
**Worse:** draft, eating.

### ℞ *Camphora officinarum* (Camphor)

**General use and quality:** sudden attacks of diarrhea where the stools are like rice water as in cholera and where the person feels extreme coldness but doesn't want to be covered up with blankets.
**Mental-Emotional:** fear at night.

### ℞ *Cantharis* (Spanish Fly)

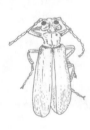

**General use and quality:** burns and sunburns where the quality of the pain is smarting, raw and burning and where the burn is swollen; and for the intense pain of second degree burns and for a blistering burn that is intensely painful.
**Mental-Emotional:** the person may be angry or irritable with the pain.
**Better:** from cold application.
**Worse:** with movement.

### ℞ *Cinchona officinalis* (Peruvian Bark–China)

**General use and quality:** dehydration, painless diarrhea with undigested food particles with lots of gas and bloating but not better from passing gas.
**General:** feels drained, exhausted from loss of fluids.
**Mental-Emotional:** apathetic and indifferent.
**Better:** bending over, warmth.
**Worse:** from loss of fluid as in diarrhea.

## *Cocculus* (Indian Cockle)

**General use and quality:** motion sickness, morning sickness, seasickness, jet lag with dizziness where everything around the person is spinning and the person experiences nausea, feels weak, trembles, with a numb empty feeling.
**Mental-Emotional:** mentally slow and lack of sleep makes time seem to pass by too fast.
**Better:** lying down.
**Worse:** from sitting, loss of sleep, or the smell of food.

## *Croton tiglium* (Croton Oil)

**General use and quality:** for skin rash due to poison ivy, poison oak, poison sumac with extremely itchy, dry red vesicles and gushing diarrhea at the same time.
**Better:** the skin feels better from applying hot water.
**Worse:** the skin feels painful from scratching.

## *Cuprum metallicum* (Copper)

**General use and quality:** for heat exhaustion where the person feels weak, faint, and nauseous with possible excessive clammy sweat and coldness of body, convulsions or jerking of muscles; diarrhea with cramps in extremities, abdomen, or calves as in cholera (one of the main remedies for cholera) where there may be nausea or retching.
**Mental-Emotional:** mental slowness, delirium.
**Better:** drinking cold water.
**Worse:** from vomiting.

## *Gelsemium* (Yellow Jasmine)

**General use and quality:** fear of an upcoming event (e.g. speaking, flying) with diarrhea from anticipation, trembling, fatigue and weakness, dullness, dizziness, drowsiness, headache; jet lag.
**Mental-Emotional:** anticipatory nervousness.
**Better:** sweating, from alcohol, from stimulants.
**Worse:** worry, sun, heat, damp weather, humidity.

**℞** *Glonoin* **(Nitroglycerine)**

> **General use and quality:** heat exhaustion and heatstroke where the headache is throbbing or pulsating, the face is hot, and the skin is sweaty.
> **Mental-Emotional:** The person is confused and irritable.
> **Better:** open air.
> **Worse:** sun, movement.

**℞** *Hypericum* **(St John's Wort)**

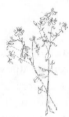

> **General use and quality:** injuries to nervous tissues such as tips of fingers, toes, tailbone (coccyx), tongue, teeth, spine; for crushing injuries to fingertips where the pain is sharp and shooting.
> **Better:** leaning backwards.
> **Worse:** stuffy rooms, getting cold.

**℞** *Kali muraticum* **(Potassium Chloride a.k.a. Tissue Salt)**

> **General use and quality:** eustachian tube and middle ear infection, fluid in the ear, plugged ear, nose and throat infetions with stringy discharge.
> **Better:** from cold drinks, from rubbing the area.
> **Worse:** in fresh air, in damp weather.

**℞** *Ledum* **(Marsh Tea)**

> **General use and quality:** inflamed and swollen bites, stings and wounds, puncture wounds where the affected part feels cold and numb; black eye where the person feels chilly.
> **Better:** wound feels better from applying ice.
> **Worse:** from heat or being heated.

**℞** *Natrum muraticum* **(Rock Salt)**

> **General use and quality:** diarrhea with sudden urgency, head blow with a headache that feels like hammers inside the head.

**General symptoms:** person is chilly but does not like the heat.
**Mental-Emotional:** serious, easily offended.
**Better:** fresh air.
**Worse:** in sun, stuffy rooms, 9–11 a.m.

### *Natrum sulfuricum* (Sodium Sulfate)

**General use and quality:** head injury from a blow to the head.
**General symptoms:** headache after head injury, sensitive to light.
**Mental-Emotional:** depression after head injury.
**Better:** fresh air.
**Worse:** damp, humid weather, lying on back.

### *Nux vomica* (Poison Nut)

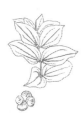

**General use and quality:** motion sickness with queasiness, chills, and possible headache at the back of the head or over one eye; constipation with constant ineffectual urging for stool, worse after alcohol.
**General symptoms:** person feels chilly, is very sensitive to light, noise, odors.
**Mental-Emotional:** irritable and oversensitive.
**Worse:** from food, tobacco smoke, and coffee.

### *Phosphorus* (Elemental Phosphorus)

**General use and quality:** for a nosebleed that will not stop where the blood is bright red and will not clot easily and the person is chilly and wants ice cold drinks but vomits them.
**Mental-Emotional:** the person is very fearful.
**Better:** from sleep, being massaged.
**Worse:** from exertion, on left side.

### *Podophyllum* (May-apple)

**General use and quality:** diarrhea that is urgent, profuse, explosive, and foul smelling; there may be gurgling before stool and the stool may be yellow, mucous filled, or bloody; the abdominal pain is generally cramping and sore, but there may be painless diarrhea.

**Mental-Emotional:** mental slowness.

**Better:** abdominal pains better from bending over, holding abdomen, after stool.

**Worse:** abdominal pains worse before or during stool.

## ℞ *Pulsatilla* (Windflower)

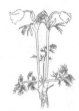

**General use and quality:** acute earaches, earaches in airplanes.

**General:** thirst-less.

**Mental-Emotional:** tearfulness, moodiness, shyness, wants attention, clingy.

**Better:** in open air.

**Worse:** in a stuffy room.

## ℞ *Rhus toxicodendron* (Poison Ivy)

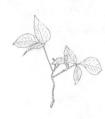

**General use and quality:** for sprains and strains where the joint is hot and swollen and there is stiffness of the joint when it is first moved and then after a while it limbers up and is better after continued motion, but worse with prolonged use. Also for the relief of poison ivy, poison oak, poison sumac with extremely itchy, red vesicles.

**Mental-Emotional:** restlessness from pain, where the person constantly moves around.

**Better:** the injury is better from heat.

**Worse:** pain is worse in cold damp weather.

## ℞ *Ruta graveolens* (Rue Bitterwort)

**General use and quality:** for sprains and strains, injuries to cartilage and tendons lying over a bone and around joints, pulled tendons and ligaments where the quality of pain is stiff and bruised.

**Better:** with movement

**Worse:** the pain is worse in wet and cold weather, and with rest.

## *Symphytum officinalis* (Comfrey)

> **General use and quality:** black eyes, blunt injury to eye, pain of eyeball; fracture to speed healing once bones are set.

## *Tabaccum* (Tobacco)

> **General use and quality:** motion sickness with nausea, dizziness and faintness, chills, sweating, sensation of a band around the head.
> **General symptoms:** person may be pale and icy cold.
> **Mental-Emotional:** disconnected.
> **Worse:** near tobacco smoke.

## *Urtica urens* (Stinging-Nettle)

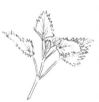

> **General use and quality:** insect bites and stings and a first degree burn with red skin but no blistering where there may be a prickly, burning feeling.
> **Better:** rubbing the area
> **Worse:** the person feels generally worse in cold, damp weather.

## *Veratrum album* (White Hellebore)

> **General use and quality:** profuse watery diarrhea which is simultaneous with vomiting (a main remedy in cholera); possible state of collapse with progressive weakness and fainting and internal icy coldness with a desire for cold water; possible profuse cold sweat especially on the forehead.
> **Better:** from lying down.
> **Worse:** cold drinks, at night.

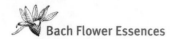 

# Bach Flower Essences

The Bach flower essences come in a water-alcohol form and you can make a dilution with 2 ounces of water and 3 drops of the tincture, then shake the dilution or cover and pound it on your hand to mix it. Bach flower remedies are safe to use and can be given for as long as the emotions persist. A usual dose is one dropper full of diluted flower essence 3 times a day.

There are specific essences prescribed for special emotional indications or states, such as honeysuckle for homesickness, but the best Bach flower remedy for the first aid kit is a combination of essences called "Rescue Remedy."

| Bach Flower Single Essences | Indication/Emotion |
|---|---|
| Clematis | drowsy, forgetful |
| Cherry Plum | fear of losing control |
| Honeysuckle | homesickness, living in the past |
| Impatiens | impatient, irritated |
| Rock Rose | fear, dread |
| Star of Bethlehem | sudden fright |

℞ **Bach Flower Combination Remedy (Rescue Remedy®)**

**Constituents:** This is a combination of cherry plum, clematis, impatiens, rock rose, and star of Bethlehem.
**Indications:** nervousness, trembling, anxiety, fear, panic, apprehension.

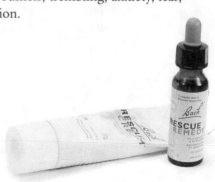

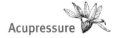

# Acupressure

According to traditional Chinese medicine theory, human energy moves through the body along pathways called meridians which surface at specific points on the body. When stimulated, these acupressure points help energy flow more evenly along meridians to balance the organs, cells, and tissues of the body. Each pressure point has been named, such as Sea of Energy for the point just below the belly button, on the conception vessel, and given a code, CV6 in this case.

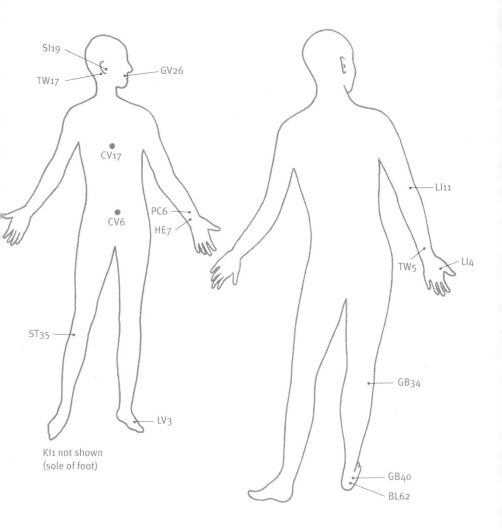

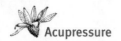 

Acupressure treatment is a method of stimulating acupuncture points with the use of finger pressure. You can do this yourself. No equipment is needed for this treatment except your hands and instructions as to which points to press. Generally, firm pressure needs to be maintained for 2 minutes and then the pressure is gradually let go.

It is important for the patient to feel something at the point you press to ensure you are at the right spot. The pressure points may feel tender, may hurt, may tingle, or a discomfort may radiate to another location. These are all good signs that you have found the right spot. If there is a great deal of tenderness at a particular point, then, according to traditional Chinese medicine, energy is blocked in this area and this point needs treatment in the way of firm pressure.

The following description of acupressure point locations and indications provide the basic knowledge for anyone to practice this form of first aid treatment. Acupressure can even be performed on oneself as needed.

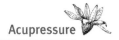

# Acupressure Points for First Aid Conditions

### Bladder 62 (BL62): Calm Sleep

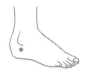

**Location:** in a depression below the outer ankle bone.
**Point indication:** relieves foot and ankle pain.
**How to perform:** press and hold for two minutes and gently release.

### Conception Vessel 6 (CV6): Sea of Energy

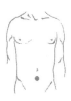

**Location:** three finger widths below the belly button in the midline of the body.
**Point action and indication:** relieves constipation and gas.
**How to perform:** lie down on back and press firmly 1–1½ inches into the abdomen or until you feel something hard for 2 minutes then gradually release.

### Conception Vessel 17 (CV17): Sea of Tranquility

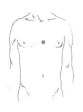

**Location:** three finger widths up from the joining of the rib cage on the breastbone in the midline of the body.
**Point action and indication:** relieves anxiety, nervousness, sensation of fullness in the chest. Helps deep breathing.
**How to perform:** measure three finger widths up from base of joining of rib cage. Press firmly and hold, taking deep breaths for two minutes.

### Gall Bladder 34 (GB34): Sunny Side of the Mountain

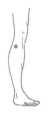

**Location:** in a depression on the outer side of the lower leg and in front of the outer bone protrusion.
**Point indication:** relieves muscle strains, knee pain.
**How to perform:** press and hold for 2 minutes and gently release. If it is too painful to firmly press this point, then rub or hold it for 30 seconds at a time.

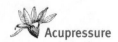 

### ℞ Gall Bladder 40 (GB40): Wilderness Mound

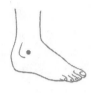

**Location:** in a depression in front of the outer ankle bone.

**Point indication:** Relieves pain and benefits tendons and ligaments.

**How to perform:** hold the point for two minutes with firm pressure then let go and repeat often.

### ℞ Heart 7 (HE7): Spirit Gate

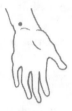

**Location:** on the wrist crease on the inner side of the tendon closest to the little finger.

**Point action and indication:** relieves anxiety, nervousness, fear.

**How to perform:** breathe deeply as you press firmly and hold for two minutes. You may feel a more sharp or radiating feeling at this point.

### ℞ Governing Vessel 26 (GV26): Middle of a Person

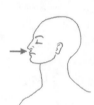

**Location:** between the upper lip and base of the nose, closer to the nose.

**Point indication:** dizziness, fainting, extreme emotional upset.

**How to perform:** firmly press between lip and base of nose for 1–2 minutes.

### ℞ Kidney 1 (KI1): Gushing Spring

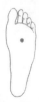

**Location:** in the center width on the sole of the foot, one third of the way from the toes to the heels.

**Point indication:** emotional shock, fainting, extreme emotional upset.

**How to perform:** press firmly for 1 minute.

### ℞ Large Intestine 4 (LI4): Joining the Valley

**Location:** in the web between the thumb and index finger at the high point of the muscle when the thumb is next to the index finger.

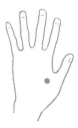

**Caution:** do not use if pregnant because it may cause contractions of the uterus.
**Point indication:** constipation, headaches.
**How to perform:** firmly squeeze in the web for 2 minutes then gently let go; change hands and repeat on opposite hand (you may feel tenderness or pain at this point); squeeze firmly enough to cause tenderness but not extreme pain.

## Large Intestine 11 (LI11): Crooked Pond

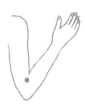

**Location:** At the end of the elbow crease on the outer edge.
**Point action and indication:** relieves constipation; stimulates the colon.
**How to perform:** place one hand on shoulder and with thumb of the other hand, apply pressure at the outer elbow crease; squeeze for 1 minute then switch hands and repeat with the opposite elbow.

## Liver 3 (LV3): Bigger Rushing

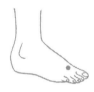

**Location:** in the webbing on top of the foot between the big toe and the second toe 2 finger widths above the crease of these 2 toes.
**Point indications:** nausea.
**How to perform:** locate the point by placing index and middle fingers together to measure from the crease of the web of the toes up two finger widths to the point; use your index finger to press firmly enough to cause tenderness to your tolerance; hold for 1 minute then repeat with other foot.

## Pericardium 6 (PC6): Inner Gate

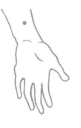

**Location:** in the center of the inner side of the forearm 3 finger widths above the wrist crease.
**Point indications:** wrist pain, nausea, travel sickness, morning sickness.
**How to perform:** press and hold for 2 minutes and gently release. If it is too painful to firmly press this point, then rub or hold it for 30 seconds at a time. Repeat whenever you feel nausea.

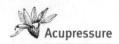 

### ℞ Small Intestine 19 (SI19): Listening Place

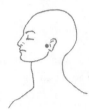

**Location:** in front of the opening to the ear. When the jaw is moved up and down, an indentation can be felt.
**Point indication:** relieves pressure inside the ear, earaches, toothaches.
**How to perform:** Press gently and make small circles to stimulate this point with the mouth open.

### ℞ Stomach 35 (ST35): Calf's Nose

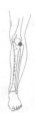

**Location:** in the depression on the outer side below the kneecap.
**Point indication:** relieves knee stiffness and pain.
**How to perform:** press and hold for 2 minutes and gently release. If it is too painful to firmly press this point, then rub or hold ift for 30 seconds at a time.

### ℞ Triple Warmer 5 (TW5): Outer Pass

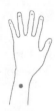

**Location:** three finger widths up from the outer wrist crease between two bones on backside of the forearm.
**Point indication:** injury to tendons, wrist pain.
**How to perform:** press and hold for 2 minutes and gently release. If it is too painful to firmly press this point, then rub or hold ift for 30 seconds at a time.

### ℞ Triple Warmer 17 (TW17): Wind Screen

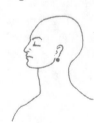

**Location:** behind the earlobe.
**Point indication:** relieves toothache and ear pain.
**How to perform:** press gently and make circular motions to stimulate this point with your fingers.

# Contents of a Naturopathic First Aid Kit

B

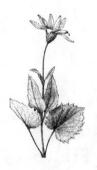

# Contents of a
# Naturopathic First Aid Kit

WHILE THERE ARE A GREAT MANY NATUROPATHIC REMEDIES and treatments for first aid conditions, they do not all need to be included in a basic first aid kit. What follows here is a list of recommended contents for a basic kit, options that provide the same or similar function so that you can choose according to conditions and availability of certain products at your local stores. The basic first aid kit can be augmented as you see fit. Besides the basic kit, the contents of several customized kits are listed. With the basic naturopathic first aid kit assembled and perhaps customized for a specific application or activity, you are ready to administer remedies for minor first aid conditions.

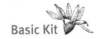

# Basic Kit

### Dressings & Accessories

- 10–20 small adhesive bandages, 3 by 1–1½ inch
- sterile gauze: one roll or 10–20 large, 4 by 4 inch, individually wrapped gauze pads.
- scissors
- tweezers
- 1 roll of adhesive tape
- cold pack
- 10–20 alcohol towlets

### Antiseptics To Clean Wounds

- Hypericum (St John's Wort) tincture, 15 ml
- Calendula tincture, 15 ml
- Tea Tree oil, 10 ml

### Cream To Promote Tissue Healing

- Calendula botanical cream, 2–4 oz
- Calendula homeopathic cream, 2–4 oz
- Vitamin E oil

### Bruising

- Arnica 30C, 80–100 pellets
- Witch Hazel distillate, 50 ml
- Arnica homeopathic cream, 2–4 oz

### Burns

- Urtica urens homeopathic ointment, 2–4 oz
- Urtica urens 30C, 20–100 pellets
- Aloe vera gel, 50 ml
- Cantharis 30C, 20–100 pellets
- Lavender essential oil

**Nerve Pain**  • Hypericum 30C, 80–100 pellets

**Fear and Upset After an Injury**

- Rescue Remedy, 10–15 ml
- Aconite 30C, 20–100 pellets
- Acupressure GV26, KI1, HE7, CV17

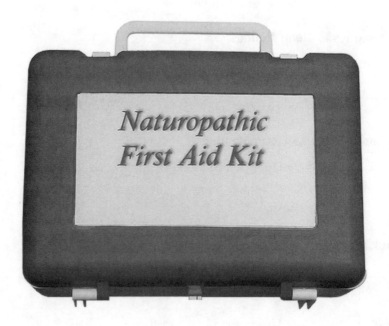

*Naturopathic First Aid Kit*

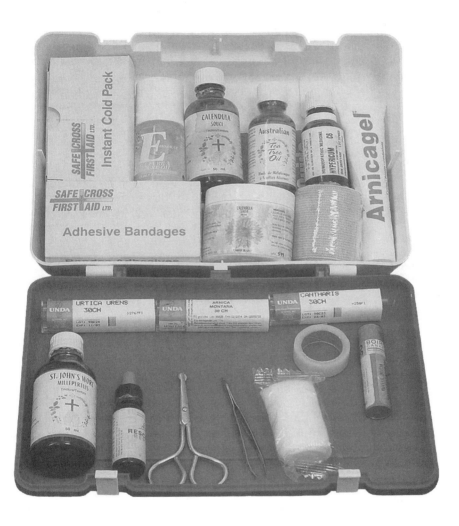

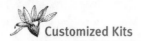 

# Customized Kits

For specific activities, the basic naturopathic first aid kit can be modified and augmented to meet the need. Here are a few customized kits. With a little study and experience, you will be able to customize your own. Many of the major suppliers of naturopathic and homeopathic remedies have likewise customized preparations and compounds for specific needs, such as ointments for soothing insect stings. To order these preparations, consult the list of suppliers at the end of the book.

## Automobile Kit (for Motion Sickness)

**Herbs:**
- Crystallized Ginger, 20–40 pieces
- Peppermint tincture, 15–30 ml or 6 tsp dried herb, sealed in a plastic bag or tea bags

**Homeopathic Remedies:**
- Cocculus 30C, 20–80 pellets
- Nux vomica 30C, 20–80 pellets
- Tabacum 30C, 20–80 pellets

**Acupressure:**
- PC6, LV3

## Cottage/Outdoors Kit
(for Insect Bites, Heat Exhaustion, and Sunburn)

**Insect Deterrent:**
- Citronella essential oil, 15 ml
- Brand name insect repellants listed in 'Naturopathic Medicine Suppliers Directory' at the back of this book.

**Topical Oil:**
- Tea Tree oil, 15 ml

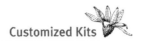

## Topical Ointments
## (for soothing Insect Bites from mosquitos and blackflies):

- Apis gel, 5–10 oz
- Tea Tree oil, 15 ml
- Lavender essential oil, 10–15 ml

## Homeopathic Remedies (for Insect Stings):

- Apis 30C (do not take below 30C during pregnancy), 20–80 pellets
- Ledum 30C, 20–80 pellets
- Carbolic acid 30C, 20–80 pellets

## Homeopathic Remedies (for Heat Exhaustion or Heat Stroke):

- Belladonna 30C, 20–80 pellets
- Bryonia 30C, 20–80 pellets
- Glonoin 30C, 20–80 pellets

## Herbal & Homeopathic Remedies (for Sunburn):

**Topical:**
- Aloe vera gel, 5–20 oz
- Lavender essential oil, 10–15 ml
- Urtica urens homeopathic cream, 10 oz
- Myoderm Homeopathic Cream (by NF Formulas Inc.), 10 oz

**Oral:**
- Belladonna 30C, 20–80 pellets
- Cantharis 30C, 20–80 pellets

# Sports Kit (for Bruising, Sprains & Strains)

## Tinctures and Ointments:

- Arnica tincture, 15–30 ml (do not apply to broken skin), or
- Arnica homeopathic cream, 5–10 oz (do not apply to broken skin)

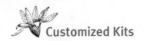 

**Homeopathic Remedies:**

- Arnica 30C, 20–80 pellets
- Bryonia 30C, 20–80 pellets
- Ruta graveolens, 30C 20–80 pellets
- Rhus toxicodendron 30C, 20–80 pellets

**Acupressure**
- BL62, GB40, GB34,
  ST35, PC6, TW5

# Travel Kit
(for Fear of Flying, Earaches, Motion Sickness, Etc)

**Fear of Flying**

**Homeopathic Remedies:**
- Aconite 30C, 20–80 pellets
- Arsenicum 30C, 20–80 pellets
- Argentum nitricum 30C, 20–80 pellets
- Gelsemium 30C, 20–80 pellets

**Bach Flower**
- Rescue Remedy

**Acupressure**
- CV17, HE17

**Earaches**

**Homeopathic Remedies:**
- Pulsatilla 30C, 20–80 pellets
- Belladonna 30C, 20–80 pellets

**Acupressure**
- TW17, SI19

**Jet Lag**

**Homeopathic Remedies:**
- Arnica 30C, 20–80 pellets
- Cocculus 30C, 20–80 pellets
- Gelsemium 30C, 20–80 pellets

**Homesickness**

**Bach Flower Essence:**
- Honeysuckle, 5–10 ml

## Motion Sickness

**Acupressure:**
- PC6, LV3

**Herbs:**
- Crystallized Ginger, 20–40 pieces
- Peppermint tincture, 15–30 ml, dried leaves 5–10 tsp

**Homeopathic Remedies:**
- Cocculus 30C, 20–80 pellets
- Nux vomica 30C, 20–80 pellets
- Tabacum 30C, 20–80 pellets

## Traveler's Diarrhea

**Rehyrating Tonic:**
- Salt, 20 g
- Baking Soda, 15 g
- Potassium Chloride, 9 g
- Glucose 120 g
- Water, 6 liters

These components are the materials that need to be mixed with water in exact proportions to make a solution high in electrolytes (salts) that are often needed when fluid is lost rapidly by the body. For a detailed explanation of how to make the solution see the travel section on diarrhea.

**Botanicals:**
- Citricidal Liquid Concentrate, 7 oz, or
- Nutribiotic Liquid Grapefruit Seed Extract, 7 oz
- Fennel seeds, 12 tsp
- Peppermint, 12 heaping tsp
- Bilberry, 90 tbsp
- Goldenseal, 30–60 ml
- Normal intestinal bacteria lactobacillus acidophilus and bifidus capsules, 1 container, 30–60 caps

**Homeopathic Remedies:**
- Arsenicum 30C, 20–80 pellets
- Camphor 30C, 20–80 pellets
- China 30C, 20–80 pellets
- Cuprum 30C, 20–80 pellets

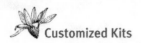 

- Natrum muraticum 30C, 20–80 pellets
- Podophyllum 30C, 20–80 pellets
- Veratrum 30C, 20–80 pellets

## Traveler's Constipation

**Acupressure:**
- LI 4, LI 11, CV6

**Homeopathic Remedies:**
- Nux vomica 30C, 20–80 pellets

# Minor First Aid Conditions

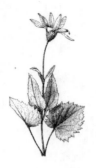

# Minor First Aid Conditions

Minor first aid conditions you can treat with your basic and customized kits are listed alphabetically in this section of the book. The symptoms of the condition are first described so that you can distinguish between minor and serious injuries and illnesses, then primary treatments are recommended, followed by secondary treatments. Primary treatment must be administered immediately and you can follow-up with secondary treatment that fits the particular symptoms of the injured or ill person.

As a rule, when a homeopathic medicine is needed, take 1 dose (3 small pellets) first by placing them under the tongue and letting them dissolve. Then use the guidelines given for how often and what dose to give. In general, if there is improvement, you do not need to take another dose of the homeopathic medicine. It is time to give another dose of the homeopathic medicine or change to a different medicine when the symptoms return or a full recovery is not reached.

# Bruising

## About Bruising (due to injury)

A bruise is bleeding under an unbroken skin surface. Tiny blood vessels break, blood leaks into the surrounding tissue and slight swelling can occur from the blood entering new spaces. The injury to tissue causes either blue or purple discoloration. As the blood gets re-absorbed the color of the bruise often changes to green or yellow. This change in the bruise color is a good sign indicating that the body is healing. Because the extent of bruising depends partly on how fragile the blood vessels are, you can minimize your bruising potential by increasing antioxidants in the diet. Particularly vitamin C and bioflavanoids (pigments found in plants) such as rutin, hesperidin, and those found in citrus peel can help to prevent bruising by minimizing capillary fragility. Bruising can be the result of other more serious conditions, such as hemophilia or certain cancers, if it is not the result of local injury. Seek medical attention if you have bruising other than from injury.

**Minor:** a banged or bumped area on arms and legs.

**Serious:** a blow to the head — refer to first aid manual and do not move someone with a serious blow to the head or spine until medical help arrives (911). Severe blow to the neck, chest, abdomen, back, groin area also requires immediate medical attention due to risk of internal bleeding. Fracture on arm or leg with associated bruising — get emergency medical attention.

**Caution:** bruising can be caused by many factors other than trauma or local tissue injury. Anemia, vitamin C deficiency, bioflavinoid deficiency, certain cancers, and the use of anticoagulant drugs can make someone bruise more easily. If you have a tendency to bruise easily, consult a health care practitioner to find the underlying cause.

## Primary Treatment

℞ **Cold Water Compress**

>Soak a towel in cold water and wrap around ice. Apply to bruised area.

℞ **Homeopathic Arnica**

>Administer Arnica 30C (3 small pellets under tongue) every 30–60 minutes for up to 4 doses.

## Secondary Treatment

℞ **Arnica Cream**  Apply arnica homeopathic or botanical cream (do not apply to broken skin)

*or*

℞ **Traumeel Ointment**

>Apply Traumeel Ointment (by Heel)

*or*

℞ **Myoderm Homeopathic Cream**

>Apply Myoderm Homeopathic Cream (by NF Formulas Inc.)

*or*

℞ **Compress of Witch Hazel (Hamamelis virginiana) or Arnica tincture**

>Apply a cold compress of a cold water soaked in a small towel with a solution of 30 drops of witch hazel herbal tincture (hamamelis virginiana) *or* 30 drops of arnica herbal tincture (do not apply to broken skin) to reduce swelling and soreness.

# Follow-up Treatment

## Homeopathic Arnica

Administer Arnica 30C (3 small pellets under tongue) twice a day, up to 5 days, until bruising is reduced. Discontinue homeopathic remedy when symptoms improve.

## Vitamin C (Ascorbic Acid)

**Form:** tablet, capsule, powder.
**Action:** promotes formation of collagen and elastin in skin, antioxidant, helps to prevent bruising.
**Indications:** bruising, burns and scalds, insect bites and stings, nosebleeds, poison ivy, scrapes, sprains and strains, sunburn.
**Dose:** 500 mg, 4 times a day with food for 2–4 weeks.
**Caution:** chewable vitamin C can damage tooth enamel and lead to cavity formation. Do not exceed 4,000 mg of vitamin C if pregnant. Do not combine with aspirin as stomach irritation or ulceration may occur.

## Bioflavanoids (rutin, hesperetin, hesperidin, quercetin)

**Form:** tablet, capsule (usually found together in a vitamin with vitamin C).
**Action:** reduces capillary fragility, antioxidant.
**Indications:** bruising, burns and scalds, insect bites and stings, nosebleeds, poison ivy, scrapes, sprains and strains, sunburn.
**Dose:** 1000 mg per day.
**Caution:** very high doses may cause diarrhea.

# Burns and Scalds (Minor)

## About Burns and Scalds

A burn is heat damaged skin. There are several types of burns classified according to their severity. A first degree burn is the least serious and only the surface is affected.

| | Type of Burn | Description | Type of Treatment |
|---|---|---|---|
| **MINOR** | **1st degree burn** | • skin pink to red<br>• feels hot to touch<br>• dry<br>• slight swelling | Topical and Homeopathy |
| **SERIOUS** | **2nd degree burn** | • red with blisters<br>• raw skin<br>• extreme pain | Homeopathy and seek medical attention. Do not apply topical treatment. |
| | **3rd degree burn** | • severe burn<br>• may have little or no pain<br>• pearly white to black skin | Seek emergency medical attention. Do not apply topical treatment. |

**Caution:** Seek emergency medical treatment for any burn that presents the following symptoms:

- swelling or blistering, especially where blisters open
- fever, nausea, chills
- burn is bigger than the size of the palm of the hand
- burn interferes with breathing
- burn is at a skin bend
- burn is electrical or chemical in origin
- the person is under age 2 or over 50 years

# Primary Treatment

### For 1st, 2nd, 3rd Degree Burn:

**Cold Water**     Immediately place the affected part under cold water.

**Homeopathic Arnica montana (Leopard's Bane)**

> **Quality:** the part feels sore.
> **Mental-Emotional:** mental shock after an injury or accident and the person may say there is nothing wrong even after a serious injury.
> **Dose:** Arnica 30C (3 small pellets under tongue) to reduce swelling and speed healing.

# Secondary Treatment

### For 1st Degree Burn only:

**Homeopathic Urtica Ointment**

> Apply to sooth superficial burns.

*or*

**Witch Hazel (Hamamelis virginiana)**

> Apply a cold compress soaked in cold water and add 1–3 tsp of witch hazel.

*or*

**Aloe vera**     Apply the gel from the inside of an aloe vera plant.

*or*

**Lavender Oil**     Apply 2–3 drops of lavender oil in 1 tsp of carrier oil such as almond oil *or* mix 2–3 drops lavender oil in aloe vera gel.

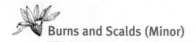 

*If the pain is not relieved by the ointment or these topical solutions, then choose either:*

**(Rx) Homeopathic Urtica urens (Stinging–nettle)**

> **General quality:** for a first degree burn with red skin but no blistering. There may be a prickly, burning feeling.
> **Dose:** Urtica urens 30C (3 small pellets under tongue) every 10 minutes or until the pain subsides, up to 5 doses. Discontinue homeopathic when symptoms improve.

*or*

**(Rx) Homeopathic Cantharis (Spanish Fly)**

> **General quality:** the quality of the pain is smarting, raw, and burning. The burn is swollen.
> **Mental-Emotional:** the person may be angry or irritable with the pain.
> **Better:** from cold application.
> **Dose:** Cantharis 30C (3 small pellets under tongue) every 10 minutes or until the pain subsides, up to 5 doses. Discontinue homeopathic when symptoms improve.

*and*

**(Rx) Vitamin E Oil** Use vitamin E oil to help heal the burn after the pain has subsided or break open a vitamin E capsule of 200 or 400 IU and apply the liquid to the burn.

### For 2nd Degree Burn:

**(Rx) Homeopathic Cantharis (Spanish Fly)**

> Use as above.

*or*

**Homeopathic Urtica urens (Stinging–nettle)**

Use as above.

## For 3rd Degree Burn:

Get medical attention immediately.

# Follow-up Treatment

**Vitamin A**　　**Form:** capsule, tablet.
**Action:** growth and repair of new tissue, antioxidant, enhances immunity.
**Indications:** burns and scalds, poison plants, scrapes, sunburn
**Dose:** 10,000 IU, 3 times a day for 2 weeks.
**Caution:** not to be taken over 10,000 IU if pregnant or you have liver disease. Vitamin A can be toxic if taken in large doses for extended periods.

**Vitamin C (Ascorbic Acid)**

**Form:** tablet, capsule, powder.
**Action:** promotes formation of collagen and elastin in skin, antioxidant, helps to prevent bruising.
**Indications:** bruising, burns and scalds, insect bites and stings, nosebleeds, poison ivy, scrapes, sprains and strains, sunburn.
**Dose:** 500 mg, 4 times a day with food for 2–4 weeks.
**Caution:** chewable vitamin C can damage tooth enamel and lead to cavity formation. Do not exceed 4,000 mg of vitamin C if pregnant. Do not combine with aspirin as stomach irritation or ulceration may occur.

**Rx Vitamin E**

**Form:** internally, capsules; topically, break open a capsule or apply oil from a container.

**Action:** antioxidant, facilitates tissue repair, reduces scarring, strengthens capillaries.

**Indications:** burns and scalds, scrapes, sunburn

**Dose:** 400 IU internally. Topically apply a thin layer of oil to affected area.

**Caution:** internally, vitamin E in large doses can elevate blood pressure. Do not take large doses of vitamin E (over 1000 IU) if on blood thinners.

**Contraindication:** externally, do not use immediately on 2nd or 3rd degree burns until the top layer of skin is healing over.

**Rx Mineral Zinc**

**Form:** tablet, capsule.

**Action:** antioxidant, repair of tissue especially for collagen formation in skin and protein synthesis.

**Indications:** burns and scalds, poison ivy, scrapes, sunburn.

**Dose:** 30 mg per day for 2–4 weeks.

**Caution:** zinc supplements can cause nausea if taken in doses higher than 30 mg at one time. Do not take more than 100 mg of zinc per day.

**Note:** poor wound healing is one sign of deficiency of zinc.

**Rx Bioflavanoids (rutin, hesperetin, hesperidin, quercetin)**

**Form:** tablet, capsule (usually found together in a vitamin with vitamin C).

**Action:** reduces capillary fragility, antioxidant.

**Indications:** bruising, burns and scalds, insect bites and stings, nosebleeds, poison ivy, scrapes, sprains and strains, sunburn.

**Dose:** 1000 mg per day.

**Caution:** very high doses may cause diarrhea.

## Essential Fatty Acids
### (from black currant oil, flax seed oil, evening primrose oil)

**Form:** capsules.

**Action:** needed for repair of cells.

**Indications:** burns and scalds, poison ivy, scrapes, sunburn.

**Dose:** 1000 mg, 3 times a day with food.

**Caution:** consult your naturopathic doctor before taking if you are on anti-clotting medication (blood thinners).

**Note:** a deficiency of essential fatty acids may be a cause of poor wound healing.

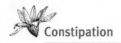 

# Constipation

## About Constipation

This is characterized by stool that is less frequent than normal or hard to pass. The stool may be hard and dry. Constipation can be caused by a lack of exercise or improper eating habits, including too many refined, processed foods, insufficient fluids or fiber. When traveling, ensure you are drinking 6–8 glasses of water a day, get regular exercise, and choose high fiber foods such as beans, fruit, vegetables, and whole grains. Any serious changes in bowel habits should be checked with a doctor.

**Minor:** stool that is difficult to pass, or not every day.

**Serious:** this condition is serious if these symptoms or signs are present:

- constipation with pain in the abdomen
- bleeding with the stool
- constipation which lasts more than five days

**Caution:** seek medical attention if constipation is serious.

## Primary Treatment

℞ **Acupressure Conception Vessel 6 (CV6): Sea of Energy**

**Point action and indication:** relieves constipation and gas.
**Location:** three finger widths below the belly button in the midline of the body.
**How to perform:** lie down on your back and press firmly 1–1½ inches into the abdomen for 2 minutes, then gradually release.

*and*

℞ **Acupressure Large Intestine 4 (LI4): Joining the Valley**

**Caution:** do not use if pregnant because it may cause contractions of the uterus.
**Point action and indication:** constipation, headaches.

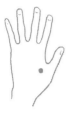

**Location:** in the web between the thumb and index finger at the high point of the muscle when the thumb is brought close to the index finger.

**How to perform:** firmly squeeze in the web for 2 minutes then gently let go. Change hands and repeat on opposite hand. You may feel tenderness or pain at this point. Squeeze firmly enough to cause tenderness to your tolerance.

*and*

## Acupressure Large Intestine 11 (LI11): Crooked Pond

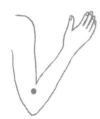

**Point action and indication:** relieves constipation. Stimulates the colon.

**Location:** at the end of the elbow crease on the outer edge.

**How to perform:** place one hand on shoulder. With the other hand, press fingers at the outer elbow crease. Squeeze for 1 minute, then switch hands and repeat with the opposite elbow.

# Secondary Treatment

## Homeopathic Nux vomica (Poison Nut)

**General use and quality:** constipation with constant ineffectual urging for stool, worse after alcohol.

**General:** person feels chilly, is very sensitive to light, noise, odors.

**Mental-Emotional:** irritable and oversensitive.

**Worse:** from food, tobacco smoke, and coffee.

**Dose:** Nux vomica 30C (3 small pellets under tongue).

# Diarrhea

## About Diarrhea

This is characterized by loose stools with increased fluid or frequency. There may be associated cramping pains. Through diarrhea, the body effectively rids itself of toxins or bacteria. Diarrhea can lead to dehydration over prolonged periods and is especially dangerous in small children and the elderly. There are many causes of diarrhea and it is important to know the cause when using herbs as treatment. For example, garlic can be used for amoebic and bacillary dysentery but not for viral diarrhea. Homeopathic remedies require that the symptoms of the person be matched to those of the remedy. The cause of the diarrhea is usually less important, unless symptoms persist for more than 24–48 hours.

The healing process involves getting rid of the invading bacteria and then allowing the natural good bacteria to re-populate the gastrointestinal tracts. Lactobacillus acidophilus, found in soured products such as plain yogurt, is a beneficial bacteria.

**Minor:** loose or frequent stools lasting less than 48 hours without blood or mucous, and without associated weakness.

**Serious:** severe or persistent (more than 48 hours) diarrhea or vomiting.

**Caution:** vomiting should last no longer than 24 hours before seeking medical attention. If you become severely weak due to dehydration or if you have persistent abdominal pain or blood in the stool, seek medical attention right away. Have children examined by a medical professional at the first signs of serious diarrhea.

# Primary Treatment

The most important treatment for diarrhea involves re-hydration, replacing the lost fluids. This is especially important in children and the elderly. Replace fluids using water, mineral water, salty water with proper proportions of water and salt, or the herbal formula for diarrhea. Drink frequently. Avoid solid food and get lots of rest.

### Re-hydration and Anti-bacterial Fluids:

You should begin to recover within a few days of administering these fluids. If there is no change within 48 hours, seek medical attention.

**Citricidal™ Liquid Concentrate (Professional Brand)**

> **Form:** liquid concentrate.
> **Action:** antibacterial, antifungal.
> **Dose:** 3–5 drops in 5–6 oz of water, in morning to prevent traveler's diarrhea, 2–3 times daily to treat diarrhea.
> **Caution:** avoid contact with eyes. Do not use undiluted.
> **Note:** available from a naturopathic doctor or health care professional.

*or*

**Nutribiotic™ Liquid Grapefruit Seed Extract**

> **Form:** liquid concentrate.
> **Action:** antibacterial, antifungal.
> **Dose:** 5–15 drops in 5–6 oz of water, in morning to prevent traveler's diarrhea, 2–3 times daily to treat diarrhea.
> **Caution:** avoid contact with eyes. Do not use undiluted.
> **Note:** available from health food stores.

**World Health Organization Formula for Diarrhea**

> 3.5 g sodium chloride (salt)
> 2.5 g sodium bicarbonate (baking soda)
> 1.5 g potassium chloride
> 20 g glucose
> 1 liter water

## Botanical Medicines:

### ℞ Fennel Seed (Foeniculum vulgare)

> **Action:** anti-spasmodic, anti-inflammatory, appetite stimulant.
>
> **Indications:** useful for diarrhea since it helps to ease colic and gas.

### ℞ Peppermint (Mentha piperita)

> **Actions:** antispasmodic, prevents vomiting, mild anesthetic antimicrobial, promotes sweating.
>
> **Indications:** colic with gas, nausea, vomiting.
>
> **Caution:** do not give to children for more than a week, do not give to babies, and do not use if breast feeding as too much can reduce milk flow.
>
> **Contraindications:** do not use if you have a hiatal hernia.
>
> **Dose:** Make a liter of tea with 2 tsp crushed fennel seeds, and 2 heaping teaspoonful of dried peppermint leaves. Then add the salt, baking soda, potassium chloride, glucose.

# Secondary Treatment

## Botanical Medicines:

### ℞ Bilberry Berries (Vaccinium myrtillus)

> **Part used:** berries.
>
> **Actions:** anti-diarrheic, astringent, antibiotic, antiseptic.
>
> **Indications:** for diarrhea such as bacterial dysentery.
>
> **Dosage:** boil 1 tbsp berries in 1 cup of water for 10 minutes, strain and drink liquid 3–6 times a day.

*and/or*

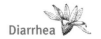

## Goldenseal (Hydrastis canadensis)

**Actions:** astringent, antispasmodic, antiseptic, antibiotic, hypoglycemic, healing to mucous membranes, reduces phlegm.

**Indications:** diarrhea, mucous conditions of respiratory or digestive tract. In vitro it has been shown to have antibiotic effects against several bacteria, protozoa, and fungi, including salmonella typhi, vibrio cholera, shigella dysenteriae, giardia lamblia.

**Dosage:** tincture 1 ml (20 drops) 3 times a day.

**Contraindication:** do not take if pregnant or lactating avoid if you have high blood pressure. In sensitive individuals, goldenseal may cause hypoglycemia (low blood sugar). Beneficial intestinal flora (lactobacillus acidophilus and bifidus) must be replaced after its use. Some people with ragweed allergies may be sensitive to goldenseal.

## Homeopathic Medicines:

## Homeopathic Arsenicum album (Arsenious Acid)

**General use and quality:** diarrhea from food poisoning, cholera. The stool is watery, acrid, especially to anus and rectum, and offensive.

**General symptoms:** burning pains, thirst for small sips of water.

**Mental-Emotional:** anxiety, nervousness, fear of death

**Better:** heat, warmth.

**Worse:** cold, being alone.

**Dose:** Arsenicum 30C (3 small pellets under tongue) after every unformed stool for up to 6 hours. If there is no effect of the remedy in 6 hours, reassess and determine if another remedy is indicated.

*or*

## Homeopathic Camphora officinarum (Camphor)

**General use and quality:** sudden attacks of diarrhea where the stools are watery and light in color, as in cholera. Extreme coldness but does not want to be covered up with blankets.

**Mental-Emotional:** fear at night.

**Dose:** Camphor 30C (3 small pellets under tongue) after every unformed stool for up to 6 hours. If there is no effect of the remedy in 6 hours, reassess and determine if another remedy is indicated.

*or*

## Homeopathic Cinchona officinalis (Peruvian Bark–China)

**General use and quality:** dehydration, painless diarrhea with undigested food particles. Lots of gas and bloating but not better from passing gas.

**General:** debilitated from loss of fluids.

**Mental-Emotional:** apathetic and indifferent.

**Better:** bending over, warmth.

**Worse:** from loss of fluid as in diarrhea.

**Dose:** China 30C (3 small pellets under tongue) after every unformed stool for up to 6 hours. If there is no effect of the remedy in 6 hours, reassess and determine if another remedy is indicated.

*or*

## Homeopathic Cuprum metallicum (Copper)

**General use and quality:** diarrhea with cramps in extremities, abdomen, or calves as in cholera (one of the main remedies for cholera). There may be nausea or retching.

**Mental-Emotional:** mental slowness, delirium.

**Better:** drinking cold water.

**Worse:** from vomiting.

**Dose:** Cuprum 30C (3 small pellets under tongue) after every unformed stool for up to 6 hours. If there is no effect of the remedy in 6 hours, reassess and determine if another remedy is indicated.

*or*

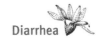

## Homeopathic Podophyllum (May-apple)

**General use and quality:** diarrhea that is urgent, profuse, explosive, and foul smelling. There may be gurgling before stool. The stool may be yellow, mucous filled, or bloody. The abdominal pain is cramping and sore. There may be painless diarrhea.
**Mental-Emotional:** mental slowness.
**Better:** abdominal pains better from bending over, holding abdomen, after stool.
**Worse:** abdominal pains worse before or during stool.
**Dose:** Podophyllum 30C (3 small pellets under tongue) after every unformed stool for up to 6 hours. If there is no effect of the remedy in 6 hours, reassess and determine if another remedy is indicated.

*or*

## Homeopathic Veratrum album (White Hellebore)

**General use and quality:** profuse watery diarrhea which is simultaneous with vomiting (a main remedy in cholera).
**General:** state of collapse with progressive weakness and possible fainting. Internal icy coldness with a desire for cold water. Simultaneous vomiting and diarrhea. There may be profuse cold sweat especially on the forehead.
**Better:** from lying down.
**Worse:** cold drinks, at night.
**Dose:** Veratrum 30C (3 small pellets under tongue) after every unformed stool for up to 6 hours. If there is no effect of the remedy in 6 hours, reassess and determine if another remedy is indicated.

## Follow-up Treatment

### ℞ Acidophilus and Lactobacillus Acidophilus

Replace friendly intestinal bacteria with lactobacillus acidophilus and lactobacillus bifidus capsules as directed on label, especially after taking goldenseal as it is antibiotic.

# Eye Injury

## About Eye Injury

An eye injury involves the eyeball or areas on the head surrounding the eye. The eye is a delicate structure because of the many blood vessels and the optic nerve which enter it, and because the lens of the eye is susceptible to scratching. The blood supply to the eye needs to be maintained in order for vision to work properly. A hemorrhage into the eyeball itself can be serious and impair vision. The optic nerve passes from the back of the eyeball through a small opening before entering the brain. In serious cases, there can be damage to the nerve or detachment of the eye from the nerve which carries visual information to the brain. Also, any swelling around the eye can put pressure on the eyeball and cause damage to the blood vessels or nerve. For all these reasons, any injury directly to the eyeball or surrounding the eye should be evaluated by a doctor. First aid measures should be undertaken only in conjunction with seeking appropriate medical evaluation and treatment.

**Minor:** no injury to the eyes is minor. See a doctor and use homeopathic medicines as needed.

**Serious:** any injury to the eye or around the eye is serious.

**Caution:** Seek emergency medical attention for

- blows causing bruising
- wounds from sharp objects
- chemicals in the eye
- any changes in vision or quality of vision

## Primary Treatment

Homeopathic Arnica montana (Leopard's Bane)

**Quality:** initial trauma of an injury. Bruising, blunt trauma to eye. The part feels sore or bruised 'as if beaten'. Everything feels too hard.

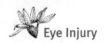

**Mental-Emotional:** mental shock after an injury or accident and the person may say there is nothing wrong even after a serious injury.
**Dose:** Arnica 30C (3 small pellets under tongue) after injury and every 4 hours, up to 5 doses. Discontinue homeopathic when symptoms improve.

## Secondary Treatment

### ℞ Homeopathic Ledum (Marsh Tea)

**Quality:** black eye where the eye feels numb and cold. The person feels chilly.
**Better:** eye feels better from applying ice.
**Worse:** from heat or being heated.
**Dose:** Ledum 30C (3 small pellets under tongue) every 4 hours up to 5 doses. Discontinue homeopathic when symptoms improve.

*or*

### ℞ Homeopathic Symphytum (Comfrey)

**Quality:** black eyes, blunt injury to eye. Pain of eyeball.
**Dose:** Symphytum 30C (3 small pellets under tongue) every 4 hours, up to 5 doses. Discontinue homeopathic when symptoms improve.

## Follow-up Treatment

### ℞ Vitamin C (Ascorbic Acid)

**Form:** tablet, capsule, powder.
**Action:** promotes formation of collagen and elastin in skin, antioxidant, helps to prevent bruising.
**Indications:** bruising, burns and scalds, insect bites and stings, nosebleeds, poison ivy, scrapes, sprains and strains, sunburn.
**Dose:** 500 mg, 4 times a day with food for 2–4 weeks.

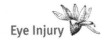

**Caution:** chewable vitamin C can damage tooth enamel and lead to cavity formation. Do not exceed 4,000 mg of vitamin C if pregnant. Do not combine with aspirin as stomach irritation or ulceration may occur.

## Bioflavanoids (rutin, hesperetin, hesperidin, quercetin)

**Form:** tablet, capsule (usually found together in a vitamin with vitamin C).

**Action:** reduces capillary fragility, antioxidant.

**Indications:** bruising, burns and scalds, insect bites and stings, nosebleeds, poison ivy, scrapes, sprains and strains, sunburn.

**Dose:** 1000 mg per day.

**Caution:** very high doses may cause diarrhea.

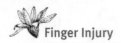 

# Finger Injury

## About Finger Injury

The fingers, toes, and tailbone are all areas of the body with lots of nerves. Because of the high concentration of nerves, crush injuries to fingers are characterized often by shooting or sharp pains and the pain may seem to radiate a distance to another part. There are two components to a crush injury: bruising or bleeding under the skin from tiny blood vessels breaking and the nerve injury. The healing process involves reducing the inflammation so the body can re-absorb the blood from the bruise, thus taking the pressure off the nerves and reducing the pain. It is important to rule out a fracture since the bones in fingers are thin. A fracture would be suspected in any case of severe pain, extensive swelling, loss of normal function, or obvious deformity. Emergency medical treatment is then necessary.

If scraped, see "Scrapes and Abrasions" (page 99). If sprained, see "Sprains and Strains" (page 103).

**Minor:** bump or bruising.

**Serious:** severe pain, loss of normal function, wounds, incisions, puncture wounds, extensive swelling, obvious deformity. Seek emergency medical treatment.

**Caution:** if pain persists, seek medical attention to determine if there is a fracture.

## Primary Treatment

### For bruising of finger:

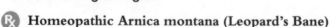 Homeopathic **Arnica montana (Leopard's Bane)**

> **Quality:** the part feels sore or bruised 'as if beaten'. Everything feels too hard.
> **Mental-Emotional:** mental shock after an injury or accident and the person may say there is nothing wrong even after a serious injury.
> **Dose:** Arnica 30C (3 small pellets under tongue) initially to reduce inflammation.

## Secondary Treatment

### For crush injuries to fingers:

### Homeopathic Hypericum (St. John's Wort)

> **Quality:** injuries to nervous tissues. Crushing injuries to fingertips. The pain is sharp and shooting.
> **Dose:** Hypericum 30C (3 small pellets under tongue) every 30–120 minutes, up to 5 doses.
> Discontinue homeopathic when symptoms improve.

## Follow-up Treatment

### Vitamin C (Ascorbic Acid)

> **Form:** tablet, capsule, powder.
> **Action:** promotes formation of collagen and elastin in skin, antioxidant, helps to prevent bruising.
> **Indications:** bruising, burns and scalds, insect bites and stings, nosebleeds, poison ivy, scrapes, sprains and strains, sunburn.
> **Dose:** 500 mg, 4 times a day with food for 2–4 weeks.
> **Caution:** chewable vitamin C can damage tooth enamel and lead to cavity formation. Do not exceed 4,000 mg of vitamin C if pregnant. Do not combine with aspirin as stomach irritation or ulceration may occur.

### Bioflavanoids (rutin, hesperetin, hesperidin, quercetin)

> **Form:** tablet, capsule (usually found together in a vitamin with vitamin C).
> **Action:** reduces capillary fragility, antioxidant.
> **Indications:** bruising, burns and scalds, insect bites and stings, nosebleeds, poison ivy, scrapes, sprains and strains, sunburn.
> **Dose:** 1000 mg per day.
> **Caution:** very high doses may cause diarrhea.

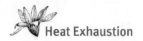 

# Heat Exhaustion

## About Heat Exhaustion

This is a condition where heavy sweating has caused a loss of fluids, affecting the circulation. Signs of dehydration may appear, such as a headache, dizziness, and blurred vision. Signs of shock may appear where there is a either a pooling of blood in dilated blood vessels in the extremities or not enough fluid in circulation. Signs of shock include cold clammy skin, shallow breathing, a fast pulse, dilated pupils, unconsciousness, and vomiting. A lack of electrolytes (salts) may cause cramps. Because heat exhaustion affects circulation to vital organs, such as the brain and heart, it is vital to find emergency medical attention, move the person out of the heat, treat the person for shock by lying in a feet up position to move more blood out of the legs and towards the heart and brain, and to replace water and salts.

Heat exhaustion is less severe than heat stroke. In heat stroke, the person has lost so much water, usually through a combination of dehydration, sweating, and sun exposure, that the body is unable to regulate temperature. This is a life-threatening situation since sweating stops and the body temperature rises quickly. Here it is vital to move the person out of the heat, cool them down, and seek emergency medical attention immediately.

**Minor:** heat exhaustion is not a minor condition. Use first aid and emergency treatment with homeopathic medicines.

**Serious:** heat stroke where the skin is hot and dry. Heat stroke is a dangerous and life-threatening condition because the body is unable to regulate temperature, sweating stops, and the body temperature increases quickly. Loss of consciousness.

**Caution:** for cases of heat exhaustion and heat stroke, call for emergency medical help immediately.

# Primary Treatment

Move the person into a shady cool place.

## If the person is conscious:

### Feet–Up Position

Treat the person for shock by lying in a feet–up position to get more blood out of the legs and towards the heart and brain.

### Saline Solution

Have the person sip on salt water with 1 tsp (5 ml) salt mixed in 1 liter or quart of water. Make sure the amount of salt is not more than this as it will make the person sick. Give as much fluid as the person will take until emergency help arrives.

## If the person is unconscious:

### Recovery Position

Lie the person down on their side and pull top knee over (recovery position). Elevate the feet.

### Monitor Symptoms

Stay with the person until emergency help arrives and monitor breathing, pulse, and other symptoms.

# Secondary Treatment

### Homeopathic Bryonia alba (Wild Hops)

**Quality:** heat exhaustion or heatstroke. There is a severe headache and may be nausea.
**Generally:** the person may feel very thirsty.
**Mental-Emotional:** the person is irritable.
**Better:** the headache is better from rest and applying something cold.

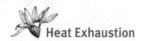 

**Worse:** the pain is worse with the slightest motion.
**Dose:** Bryonia 30 C (3 small pellets under tongue) every 5 minutes. Discontinue when symptoms improve. Follow-up 30C every 1–2 hours, up to 5 doses.

*or*

### ℞ Homeopathic Glonoin (Nitro–glycerine)

**Quality:** heat exhaustion and heat stroke. The headache is throbbing or pulsating. The face is hot and the skin is sweaty.
**Mental-Emotional:** the person is confused and irritable.
**Dose:** Glonoin 30 C (3 small pellets under tongue) every 5 minutes. Discontinue when symptoms improve. Follow-up 30C every 1–2 hours, up to 5 doses.

*or*

### ℞ Homeopathic Belladonna (Deadly Nightshade)

**Quality:** heat exhaustion or heat stroke that comes on suddenly. The person has a throbbing headache, the skin is hot and dry.
**General:** the person has a red flushed face with dilated pupils.
**Mental-Emotional:** in heat exhaustion or heatstroke, the person may be delirious, have hallucinations, or lose consciousness.
**Dose:** Belladonna 30 C (3 small pellets under tongue) every 5 minutes. Discontinue when symptoms improve. Follow-up 30C every 1–2 hours, up to 5 doses.

# Insect Bites (Mosquito, Spider, or Fly)

## About Insect Bites

Insect bites are characterized by a red area 6 mm (¼ inch) surrounding the bite area. Insect bites are uncomfortable and itchy. There is a risk of infection, especially with blackfly bites, as a small part of the skin has been removed.

Insect bites swell because the immune system recognizes the anticoagulant that the mosquito injects or blackfly secretes into the bite surface as foreign. It may take several days to two weeks for healing to occur. The bite area has less swelling as the body breaks down the wall of inflammation. How quickly an insect bite heals may depend on one's nutritional status. Adequate levels of vitamin C, zinc, and protein are essential to proper healing of the skin surface.

**Minor:** mosquito, spider, blackfly bites.

**Serious:** insect bite with lots of swelling. Signs of allergic reaction, such as swelling of the throat, hives, or difficulty breathing, weakness, headache, fever, abdominal cramps, vomiting, redness spreading from the area. At the first signs of an allergic reaction, get emergency medical attention.

**Caution:** check the insect bite every day and seek medical attention for an infected insect bite if there is increasing pain, redness, swelling, red streaks away from the injury site, foul smelling pus, or fever, chills, lymphodenopathy (swollen glands).

## Prevention

### Cover-up

Be sure to wear protective clothing. Make sure shirts are tucked into pants and pant legs are tucked into socks.

**Citronella Oil**    Apply citronella oil to exposed skin.

**Tea Tree Oil**    Apply undiluted tea tree oil to small areas of exposed skin, or for larger areas of exposed skin, use 7 drops mixed in 1 tbsp of carrier oil.

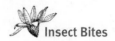 

℞ **Repellants**    Apply brand name insect repellants listed in 'Naturopathic Medicine Suppliers Directory' at the back of this book.

## Primary Treatment

### Topical applications for relief of the itch of insect bites:

℞ **Witch Hazel (Hamamelis virginiana)**

Apply a compress of witch hazel, 30 drops (1 tsp) of witch hazel on gauze.

*or*

℞ **Apis Gel**    Apply Apis gel (by Dolisos) to help relieve the itch, swelling, sting, or burning of bites.

*or*

℞ **Lavender Essential Oil**

Apply lavender essential oil, one or two drops to each bite.

*or*

℞ **St John's Wort**    Apply tincture of St. John's Wort, 2–3 drops directly to the bite area.

*If there is much swelling, these internal homeopathic medicines may be useful:*

℞ **Homeopathic Apis 30C Apis mellifica (Honey Bee)**

**Quality:** the pain is stinging and burning and there is much swelling that comes on quickly. The area feels hot to the touch. The person will not be thirsty.
**Mental-Emotional:** there may be restlessness and irritability.
**Better:** from applying cold to the area.
**Worse:** from touching or applying heat to the area.

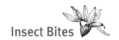

**Caution:** do not take below 30C during pregnancy (i.e., do not take X potencies or 6C or 12C).
**Dose:** Apis 30C (3 small pellets under tongue) every 2 hours to relieve the swelling, up to 5 doses. Discontinue homeopathic when symptoms improve.

*or*

### Homeopathic Ledum (Marsh Tea)

**Quality:** inflamed and swollen bites where wound feels cold and numb. The person feels chilly.
**Better:** from applying ice
**Worse:** from heat or being heated
**Dose:** Ledum 30C (3 small pellets under tongue) every 2 hours, for up to 5 doses. Discontinue homeopathic when symptoms improve.

## Follow-up Treatment

### Vitamin C (Ascorbic Acid)

**Form:** tablet, capsule, powder.
**Action:** promotes formation of collagen and elastin in skin, antioxidant, helps to prevent bruising.
**Indications:** bruising, burns and scalds, insect bites and stings, nosebleeds, poison ivy, scrapes, sprains and strains, sunburn.
**Dose:** 500 mg, 4 times a day with food for 2–4 weeks.
**Caution:** chewable vitamin C can damage tooth enamel and lead to cavity formation. Do not exceed 4,000 mg of vitamin C if pregnant. Do not combine with aspirin as stomach irritation or ulceration may occur.

### Bioflavanoids (rutin, hesperetin, hesperidin, quercetin)

**Form:** tablet, capsule (usually found together in a vitamin with vitamin C).
**Action:** reduces capillary fragility, antioxidant.

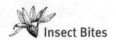 

**Indications:** bruising, burns and scalds, insect bites and stings, nosebleeds, poison ivy, scrapes, sprains and strains, sunburn.
**Dose:** 1000 mg per day.
**Caution:** very high doses may cause diarrhea.

# Insect Stings (Bees, Wasps, and Hornets)

## About Insect Stings

Stings from bees or wasps can be very painful due to the venom injected by the insect. There is usually also redness, some swelling, 6–12 mm (¼–½ inch) diameter, around the site as the body mounts an immune response to the insect sting. Stings are dangerous due to the potential of allergic reactions to the venom. When the stinger pierces the skin, venom made up of protein is injected. The immune system reacts to the proteins in the venom and can trigger an anaphylactic allergic reaction where the body's reaction is out of proportion. An anaphylactic allergy is rare but is a potential danger. Always be aware of the signs and symptoms of serious allergic reactions.

Bees can only sting once as a pouch is dislodged carrying more venom and they die upon stinging. Because of this pouch, it is important not to use tweezers to pull out stingers as this will squeeze more venom into the area. The use of a credit card or object to scrape the stinger out from the tip is the best way to prevent more venom entering the body.

The bite area has less swelling as the body breaks down the wall of inflammation. The use of cold can help to numb the area and decrease both pain and swelling. An insect sting may heal more quickly depending on one's nutritional status. Adequate levels of vitamin C, zinc, and protein are essential to proper healing of the skin surface.

**Minor:** stings with no signs of allergic reaction or infection. Do not squeeze or remove stinger with tweezers as this will force the venom out.

**Serious:** a bite with signs of allergic reaction, such as

- swelling of the throat
- hives
- difficulty breathing
- rapid pulse
- vertigo (dizziness)
- paleness
- weakness
- headache
- fever
- abdominal cramps
- vomiting
- redness spreading from the area

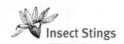 

**Caution:** at the first sign of an allergic reaction, get immediate medical help as soon as possible. Do not squeeze or remove stinger with tweezers as this will force the venom out. If a sting is inside the mouth, give the person a piece of ice to suck on or rinse mouth with 1 tsp of baking soda in a glass of water and get medical help. Administer Homeopathic Carbolic Acid 30.

## Primary Treatment ·

### If the sting shows signs of being serious:

℞ **Homeopathic Carbolic Acid**

> **Quality:** anaphylactic reaction to bee or wasp sting with swelling of face, throat, tongue. Ears feel swollen, difficulty breathing, the person is pale, with cold sweat, blisters that burn and itch.
> **General:** the person is in a state of collapse.
> **Dose:** Carbolic acid 30 (3 small pellets under tongue), 1 dose every 20 seconds until symptoms improve while on the way to or waiting for emergency medical attention.

### If minor:

℞ **Remove Stinger**

> Remove wasp or bee stinger by scraping it out with a sharp edge like a knife blade or credit card.

℞ **Ice, Ammonia, Baking Soda**

> Place ice on the sting, or ammonia, or a paste of baking soda and water to reduce pain.

## Secondary Treatment

℞ **Homeopathic Arnica montana (Leopard's Bane)**

> **Quality:** initial trauma of an injury. The part feels sore or bruised 'as if beaten'. Everything feels too hard.

**Mental-Emotional:** mental shock after an injury or accident and the person may say there is nothing wrong even after a serious injury.
**Dose:** Arnica 30C (3 small pellets under tongue).

*followed by*

## Homeopathic Ledum (Marsh Tea)

**Quality:** inflamed and swollen bites where wound feels cold and numb. The person feels chilly.
**Better:** from applying ice.
**Worse:** from heat or being heated.
**Dose:** Ledum 30C (3 small pellets under tongue) every 2 hours for up to 5 doses. Discontinue homeopathic when symptoms improve.

*or*

## Homeopathic Apis mellifica (Honey Bee)

**Quality:** the pain is stinging and burning and there is much swelling that comes on quickly. The area feels hot to the touch. The person will not be thirsty.
**Mental-Emotional:** there may be restlessness and irritability.
**Better:** from applying cold to the area.
**Worse:** from touching or applying heat to the area.
**Caution:** do not take below 30C during pregnancy (i.e., do not take X potencies or 6C or 12C).
**Dose:** Apis 30C (3 small pellets under tongue) every 2 hours to relieve the swelling, up to 5 doses. Discontinue homeopathic when symptoms improve.

*or*

## Homeopathic Carbolic Acid

**Quality:** swelling of face, throat, tongue. Ears feel swollen, difficulty breathing, the person is pale, cold sweat, blisters that burn and itch.
**Dose:** Carbolic acid 30 (3 small pellets under tongue), 1 dose every 20 seconds until symptoms improve while on the way to or waiting for emergency medical attention.

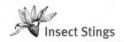 

# Follow-up Treatment

### Monitor for Infection

Check the insect sting every day and seek medical attention for an infected sting. An infection occurs when bacteria get into a broken or open area of skin and multiply. For any of the following signs it is important to seek medical attention immediately because they signal infection:

- increasing pain
- redness
- swelling
- red streaks towards the body from the injury site
- foul smelling pus
- fever

### Vitamin C (Ascorbic Acid)

**Form:** tablet, capsule, powder.

**Action:** promotes formation of collagen and elastin in skin, antioxidant, helps to prevent bruising.

**Indications:** bruising, burns and scalds, insect bites and stings, nosebleeds, poison ivy, scrapes, sprains and strains, sunburn.

**Dose:** 500 mg, 4 times a day with food for 2–4 weeks.

**Caution:** chewable vitamin C can damage tooth enamel and lead to cavity formation. Do not exceed 4,000 mg of vitamin C if pregnant. Do not combine with aspirin as stomach irritation or ulceration may occur.

### Bioflavanoids (rutin, hesperetin, hesperidin, quercetin)

**Form:** tablet, capsule (usually found together in a vitamin with vitamin C).

**Action:** reduces capillary fragility, antioxidant.

**Indications:** bruising, burns and scalds, insect bites and stings, nosebleeds, poison ivy, scrapes, sprains and strains, sunburn.

**Dose:** 1000 mg per day.

**Caution:** very high doses may cause diarrhea.

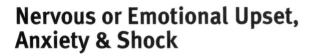

# Nervous or Emotional Upset, Anxiety & Shock

## About Nervous or Emotional Upset, Anxiety and Shock

Nervous upset after injury is the feeling of nervousness, anxiety, trembling, and worry. The experience of an accident can bring about much anxiety, but this condition differs from shock in that it is emotional in nature. It is important to be aware of the physical symptoms of shock. Shock is a serious and potentially life threatening situation where the blood is diverted away from the vital organs and pools in the extremities. For this reason, the heart has a hard time getting blood circulation to the organs and speeds up, the person appears pale and sweating with cold clammy skin, and the person may feel weak and faint. Emergency medical attention is needed and the person should be covered and placed on their side with the feet elevated. Monitor for pulse and breathing until help arrives.

**Minor:** emotional upset with no signs of shock.

**Serious:** signs of shock such as:

- paleness with sweating
- cold limbs
- rapid weak pulse
- person feels cold and clammy to the touch
- person feels weak and faint

**Caution:** if the person does show these signs of shock, call for emergency medical help, then lie the person down on their side with feet elevated. Wrap the person in a warm blanket, and monitor for pulse and breathing until emergency help arrives. This is a serious condition. If mental shock lasts for more than a few days, seek medical attention.

## Primary Treatment

**℞ Bach Flower Rescue Remedy**

> 1 dropper full of diluted tincture (2 oz water and 3 drops tincture), for nervousness and trembling worry or panic.

*or*

**℞ Homeopathic Arnica montana (Leopard's Bane)**

> **Mental-Emotional:** mental shock after an injury or accident and the person may say there is nothing wrong even after a serious injury.
> **Dose:** Arnica 30C initially after the accident.
> **Follow-up:** Arnica 30C (3 small pellets under tongue) once a day for up to 2 days. Discontinue when symptoms improve.

*or*

**℞ Homeopathic Aconite Aconitum napellus (Monkshood)**

> **Quality:** for mental shock and fear immediately after an injury or traumatic event.
> **Mental-Emotional:** anxiety and restlessness after an injury or fright.
> **Worse:** after exposure to cold dry wind.
> **Dose:** Aconite 30C initially after the accident.
> **Follow-up:** Aconite 30C (3 small pellets under tongue) once a day for up to 2 days. Discontinue when symptoms improve.

**℞ Acupressure Governing Vessel 26 (GV26): Middle of a Person**

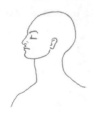

> **Location:** between upper lip and nose.
> **Point indication:** emotional upset, dizziness, fainting.
> **How to perform:** press firmly with your finger towards the gums between your upper lip and nose, for 2 minutes.

## Acupressure Kidney (KI1): Gushing Spring

**Location:** in the middle of the sole of the foot, one-third of the way from the base of the toes to the heel.
**Point indication:** dizziness, mental shock.
**How to perform:** press firmly or rub firmly for 1 minute, then switch and press or rub the other foot.

## Acupressure HE7: Spirit Gate

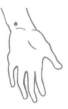

**Location:** at the wrist crease on the inner side of the tendon which is closet to the little finger.
**Point indication:** palpitations, racing heart, nervous anxiety.
**How to perform:** press and firmly hold for 1 minute, then switch to the point on the other hand, press and firmly hold.

## Acupressure Conception Vessel (CV17): Sea of Tranquility

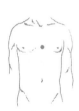

**Location:** on the middle of the breastbone, 3 inches up from the base of the bone.
**Point indication:** fear, anxiety, nervousness, heart palpitations.
**How to perform:** press and hold firmly for 2 minutes.

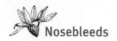 

# Nosebleeds (not from a head or spinal injury)

## About Nosebleeds

Nosebleeds are usually due to trauma to the blood vessels in the nose. The blood vessels lie close to the surface and are prone to irritation, especially in children who pick their nose frequently or those who blow too hard. The blood that comes from a nosebleed may seem profuse, and it is important to take measures to stop the bleeding. Pinching the nose helps to create pressure to stop the flow of blood. A cold compress can also be used to help stop the bleeding. A minor nosebleed should stop within 5–15 minutes. The healing process involves clotting cells to form a network and block the tear in the blood vessel. Nutritional status may contribute to reduced nosebleeds. Foods high in vitamin K help with the clotting process; some of the best sources are dark green leafy vegetables.

**Minor:** a nosebleed not from a head or spinal injury, from blowing nose too hard, for no apparent reason.

**Serious:** a blow to the head or a fall causing bleeding from the nose.

**Caution:** if you suspect a head or spinal injury (injury to the neck or back) from a blow to the head or a fall, do not move the person and do not stop the bleeding. Call for emergency medical help. If the blood from the nose is mixed with straw colored fluid or the bleeding does not stop or starts again, get medical help as soon as possible.

## Primary Treatment

**Tilt Head Forward**

Have the person sit with the head tilted forward to allow the blood to drain out.

**Pinch Nose**     Pinch gently the fleshy part of the nose just above the tip until the bleeding stops (about 10 minutes).

**Cold Cloth**     Apply a cloth or towel soaked in cold water to back of the neck and nose.

### Do Not Blow Nose

Do not blow the nose for a few hours.

# Secondary Treatment

**Note:** If a homeopathic remedy is not giving relief within 5 to 10 minutes, a different remedy may be needed.

### Homeopathic Arnica montana (Leopard's Bane)

**General use and quality:** nosebleeds from an injury or blowing the nose too hard. The part feels sore or bruised 'as if beaten'. Everything feels too hard.
**Mental-Emotional:** mental shock after an injury or accident and the person may say there is nothing wrong even after a serious injury.
**Dose:** Arnica 30C (3 small pellets under tongue) every 2 minutes for up to 3 doses.

*or*

### Homeopathic Phosphorus (Elemental Phosphorus)

**Quality:** for a nosebleed that will not stop. The blood is bright red and will not clot easily. The person is chilly and wants ice cold drinks.
**Mental-Emotional:** the person is very fearful.
**Dose:** Phosphorus 30C (3 small pellets under tongue) every 2 minutes for up to 3 doses.

*or*

### Belladonna (Deadly Nightshade)

**General use and quality:** a nosebleed that comes on suddenly. The blood is hot and clots easily.
**General:** the person has a red flushed face with dilated pupils.
**Dose:** Belladonna 30C (3 small pellets under tongue) every 2 minutes for up to 3 doses.

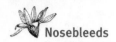 

## Follow-up Treatment

### Vitamin C (Ascorbic Acid)

**Form:** tablet, capsule, powder.

**Action:** promotes formation of collagen and elastin in skin, antioxidant, helps to prevent bruising.

**Indications:** bruising, burns and scalds, insect bites and stings, nosebleeds, poison ivy, scrapes, sprains and strains, sunburn.

**Dose:** 500 mg, 4 times a day with food for 2–4 weeks.

**Caution:** chewable vitamin C can damage tooth enamel and lead to cavity formation. Do not exceed 4,000 mg of vitamin C if pregnant. Do not combine with aspirin as stomach irritation or ulceration may occur.

# Poison Ivy, Poison Oak, Poison Sumac

## About Poison Ivy, Poison Oak, Poison Sumac

The resins contained in the roots, stems, berries, and leaves of these plants cause an allergic reaction which is more severe in some people than in others. Contact with the plant resin can cause a red, itchy rash with fluid-filled blisters if it is not washed off the skin within 10 minutes of contact. The rash may appear from a few hours after contact to a few days later and may last up to four weeks. There is usually oozing and crusting of the blisters before the skin is fully healed.

**Minor:** itchy rash, blistering, redness at the site.

**Serious:** signs of allergic reaction, such as swelling of the throat or difficulty breathing, hives, fever, abdominal cramps, vomiting, redness spreading from the area. A large surface area, pain or swelling of the genitals, pain or swelling of the face, much discomfort at the site (itchiness or pain)

**Caution:** at the first signs of allergic reaction, seek emergency medical attention. Check the area daily for infection and seek medical attention if there is increasing pain, redness, swelling, red streaks away from the injury site, foul smelling pus, fever, chills, or lymphodenopathy (swollen glands).

## Prevention

**Keep Away**

Keep away from these plants by knowing how to identify them:

Poison ivy is found throughout the United States and southern Canada. It is a shrub or vine that grows from 2–7 feet tall. The leaves are in groups of three with the end leaf on a longer stalk, and the side leaves opposite each other. There can be a white cluster of berries. The leaves may turn red in the fall.

Poison oak is more common in the western part of the United States and Canada. It has the same three-leaf pattern as poison ivy, except the leaves resemble those of an oak tree.

Poison sumac grows as a shrub or small tree with 7–13 leaves. White clusters of berries may be visible on this plant.

**Cover Up**  Wear shoes, socks, long pants to minimize skin exposure when going for a walk in the woods. Avoid touching clothing when removing if you suspect you might have brushed up against one of these poisonous plants.

## Primary Treatment

### Soap and Water

Wash contact area with soap and water as soon as possible since it takes about 10 minutes for the resin to sink in.

### Cold Compress

Apply a cold compress to the affected area.

## Secondary Treatment

### Ⓡ Calendula Tincture

Apply to the skin rash 4 or more times daily to help relieve itching and promote skin healing.

*or*

### Ⓡ Sea Salt Cold Compress

Apply a cold compress made of 1 tbsp sea salt in 1 pint water to relieve itching.

*and/or*

### Homeopathic Rhus toxicodendron (Poison Ivy)

**Quality:** extremely itchy, red vesicles.
**General:** the person may be chilly and worse from cold or dampness.
**Mental-Emotional:** restlessness.
**Worse:** the skin feels worse from heat.
**Dose:** Rhus toxicodendron 30C (3 small pellets under tongue) every few hours (or as needed) to relieve the itching.

*or*

### Homeopathic Anacardium (Marking Nut)

**Quality:** extremely itchy rash that has a yellow discharge from the blisters.
**General:** the person may be so itchy that they scratch until they bleed.
**Better:** the skin feels better from applying hot water.
**Dose:** Anacardium 30C (3 small pellets under tongue) every few hours (or as need) to relieve itching.

*or*

### Homeopathic Croton tiglium (Croton Oil)

**General use and quality:** extremely itchy, dry red vesicles and gushing diarrhea at the same time.
**Worse:** the skin feels painful from scratching.
**Dose:** Croton tiglium 30C (3 small pellets under tongue) ever few hours (or as needed) to relieve itching.

## Follow-up Treatment

**Vitamin A**
**Form:** capsule, tablet.
**Action:** growth and repair of new tissue, antioxidant, enhances immunity.
**Indications:** burns and scalds, poison plants, scrapes, sunburn.
**Dose:** 10,000 IU, 3 times a day for 2 weeks.

**Caution:** not to be taken over 10,000 IU if pregnant or you have liver disease. Vitamin A can be toxic if taken in large doses for extended periods.

## ℞ Vitamin C (Ascorbic Acid)

**Form:** tablet, capsule, powder.

**Action:** promotes formation of collagen and elastin in skin, antioxidant, helps to prevent bruising.

**Indications:** bruising, burns and scalds, insect bites and stings, nosebleeds, poison ivy, scrapes, sprains and strains, sunburn.

**Dose:** 500 mg, 4 times a day with food for 2–4 weeks.

**Caution:** chewable vitamin C can damage tooth enamel and lead to cavity formation. Do not exceed 4,000 mg of vitamin C if pregnant. Do not combine with aspirin as stomach irritation or ulceration may occur.

## ℞ Mineral Zinc

**Form:** tablet, capsule.

**Action:** antioxidant, repair of tissue especially for collagen formation in skin and protein synthesis.

**Indications:** burns and scalds, poison ivy, scrapes, sunburn.

**Dose:** 30 mg per day for 2–4 weeks.

**Caution:** zinc supplements can cause nausea if taken in doses higher than 30 mg at one time. Do not take more than 100 mg of zinc per day.

**Note:** poor wound healing is one sign of deficiency of zinc.

## ℞ Essential Fatty Acids
## (from black currant oil, flax seed oil, evening primrose oil)

**Form:** capsules.

**Action:** needed for repair of cells.

**Indications:** burns and scalds, poison ivy, scrapes, sunburn.

**Dose:** 1000 mg, 3 times a day with food.

**Caution:** consult your naturopathic doctor before taking if you are on anti-clotting medication (blood thinners).

**Note:** a deficiency of essential fatty acids may be a cause of poor wound healing.

# Scrapes and Abrasions

## About Scrapes and Abrasions

This is an injury to the surface layer of the skin from rubbing or scraping against a hard or rough surface. The skin is not spread apart, but there may be dirt in the scrape. White blood cells (immune cells) migrate to the area and some bleeding may occur. A scrape will start to resolve by forming a clotted area or scab over the area, followed by the scab falling off in 1 to 2 weeks. It is important to check the scrape every day and seek medical attention for an infected scrape. An infection occurs when bacteria get into a broken or open area of skin and multiply. For any of the following signs it is important to seek medical attention immediately because they signal infection: if there is increasing pain, redness, swelling, red streaks towards the body from the injury site, foul smelling pus, or fever.

**Minor:** the surface of the skin and blood vessels below are exposed but the skin is not spread apart. There is often dirt in a scrape. Little or no bleeding.

**Serious:** lots of dirt. Bleeding that does not stop after putting direct pressure and elevating. Wound deeper than the skin layer such as an incision, laceration, puncture wound, or wound with torn away skin.

**Caution:** seek medical attention if bleeding does not stop after putting on a sterile dressing and applying direct pressure or if objects are stuck in skin (e.g., stick, glass, rock, asphalt). Check the scrape every day and seek medical attention for an infected scrape or wound if there is increasing pain, redness, swelling, red streaks towards the body from the injury site, foul smelling pus, or fever.

## Primary Treatment

### Calendula and Hypericum

Clean cut or scrape with gauze soaked with calendula and hypericum, 5 drops of each in 1 cup of water.

*or*

Ⓡ **Calendula and Hypericum Tincture**

Clean scrape with 10 drops of calendula tincture in 1 cup of water or 10 drops of hypericum tincture in 1 cup of water.

*and*

Ⓡ **Calendula Cream**

Apply calendula cream — botanical (has antiseptic properties) or homeopathic(does not have antiseptic properties) — and cover with a sterile dressing and change as needed for 2–3 days.

*or*

Ⓡ **Tea Tree Oil**    Apply 2–3 drops of tea tree oil to scrape and cover with a sterile dressing and change as needed for 2–3 days. Caution: this may sting.

## Secondary Treatment

If the scrape is also bruised, to reduce swelling, pain, and speed healing:

Ⓡ **Homeopathic Arnica montana (Leopard's Bane)**

**Quality:** the part is bruised.
**Mental-Emotional:** mental shock after an injury or accident and the person may say there is nothing wrong even after a serious injury.
**Oral Dose:** Arnica 30C (3 small pellets under tongue). Discontinue homeopathic when symptoms improve.

Ⓡ **Vitamin E Oil**    Use vitamin E oil topically to promote healing after 2–3 days if the scrape is healing and none of the following are present: increasing pain, redness, swelling, red streaks towards the body from the injury site, foul smelling pus, or fever.

# Follow-up Treatment

**Vitamin A**

**Form:** capsule, tablet.
**Action:** growth and repair of new tissue, antioxidant, enhances immunity.
**Indications:** burns and scalds, poison plants, scrapes, sunburn
**Dose:** 10,000 IU, 3 times a day for 2 weeks.
**Caution:** not to be taken over 10,000 IU if pregnant or you have liver disease. Vitamin A can be toxic if taken in large doses for extended periods.

**Vitamin C (Ascorbic Acid)**

**Form:** tablet, capsule, powder.
**Action:** promotes formation of collagen and elastin in skin, antioxidant, helps to prevent bruising.
**Indications:** bruising, burns and scalds, insect bites and stings, nosebleeds, poison ivy, scrapes, sprains and strains, sunburn.
**Dose:** 500 mg, 4 times a day with food for 2–4 weeks.
**Caution:** chewable vitamin C can damage tooth enamel and lead to cavity formation. Do not exceed 4,000 mg of vitamin C if pregnant. Do not combine with aspirin as stomach irritation or ulceration may occur.

**Vitamin E**

**Form:** internally, capsules; topically, break open a capsule or apply oil from a container.
**Action:** antioxidant, facilitates tissue repair, reduces scarring, strengthens capillaries.
**Indications:** burns and scalds, scrapes, sunburn
**Dose:** 400 IU internally. Topically apply a thin layer of oil to affected area.
**Caution:** internally, vitamin E in large doses can elevate blood pressure. Do not take large doses of vitamin E (over 1000 IU) if on blood thinners.

**Mineral Zinc**

**Form:** tablet, capsule.
**Action:** antioxidant, repair of tissue especially for collagen formation in skin and protein synthesis.

**Indications:** burns and scalds, poison ivy, scrapes, sunburn.

**Dose:** 30 mg per day for 2–4 weeks.

**Caution:** zinc supplements can cause nausea if taken in doses higher than 30 mg at one time. Do not take more than 100 mg of zinc per day.

**Note:** poor wound healing is one sign of deficiency of zinc.

## Bioflavanoids (rutin, hesperetin, hesperidin, quercetin)

**Form:** tablet, capsule (usually found together in a vitamin with vitamin C).

**Action:** reduces capillary fragility, antioxidant.

**Indications:** bruising, burns and scalds, insect bites and stings, nosebleeds, poison ivy, scrapes, sprains and strains, sunburn.

**Dose:** 1000 mg per day.

**Caution:** very high doses may cause diarrhea.

## Essential Fatty Acids (from black currant oil, flax seed oil, evening primrose oil)

**Form:** capsules.

**Action:** needed for repair of cells.

**Indications:** burns and scalds, poison ivy, scrapes, sunburn.

**Dose:** 1000 mg, 3 times a day with food.

**Caution:** consult your naturopathic doctor before taking if you are on anti-clotting medication (blood thinners).

**Note:** a deficiency of essential fatty acids may be a cause of poor wound healing.

# Sprains and Strains

## About Sprains and Strains

This is injury to ligaments (sprains) and muscles (strains), usually caused by overuse or trauma. There may be bruising, swelling, pain around or loss of use of a joint or in a muscle. It is important to stop playing a sport as soon as you feel pain. Playing through an injury such as a sprain will make it worse and lengthen time for healing.

**Minor:** sprains or strains to limbs with normal function and minimal pain and swelling.

**Serious:** sprains and strains may be serious when these symptoms or signs as present:

- excessive swelling
- loss of function in a joint, can't stand or walk
- deformed joint or limb
- wound around the joint
- severe pain that is not going away after days
- severe blow to the neck, chest, abdomen, back, groin area with significant discoloration due to internal bleeding

**Caution:** seek medical attention immediately when sprains or strains are serious.

## Primary Treatment

### Topical:

### Arnica Tincture and Ice

Wrap ice in a damp towel soaked in 10 drops of Arnica tincture and place on the area alternating 5 minutes on and 2 minutes off. Rest, ice (as above), use compression, and elevate the affected limb.

### Oral:

(R) **Homeopathic Arnica montana (Leopard's Bane)**

> **Quality:** initial trauma of an injury. Sprains or strains with bruising. The part feels sore or bruised 'as if beaten'. Everything feels too hard.
> **Mental-Emotional:** mental shock after an injury or accident and the person may say there is nothing wrong even after a serious injury.
> **Dose:** Arnica 30C (3 small pellets under tongue) immediately after injury to reduce swelling and bruising
> **Caution:** if pain and swelling are not relieved in 1–2 days see a doctor.

### For swelling and pain from ankle sprain:

(R) **Acupressure Bladder 62 (BL62): Calm Sleep**

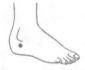

> **Location:** in a depression below the outer ankle bone.
> **Point indication:** relieves foot and ankle pain.
> **How to perform:** press and hold for two minutes and gently release.

(R) **Acupressure Gall Bladder 40 (GB40): Wilderness Mound**

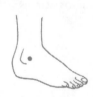

> **Location:** in a depression in front to the outer ankle bone.
> **Point indication:** Relieves pain and benefits tendons and ligaments.
> **How to perform:** hold the point for two minutes with firm pressure then let go and repeat often.

### For knee pain:

(R) **Acupressure Gall Bladder 34 (GB34): Sunny Side of the Mountain**

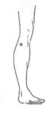

> **Location:** in a depression on the outer side of the lower leg and in front of the outer bone protrusion.
> **Point indication:** relieves muscle strains, knee pain.

**How to perform:** press and hold for 2 minutes and gently release. If it is too painful to firmly press this point, then rub or hold it for 30 seconds at a time.

## Acupressure Stomach 35 (ST35): Calf's Nose

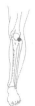

**Location:** in the depression on the outer side below the kneecap.
**Point indication:** relieves knee stiffness and pain.
**How to perform:** press and hold for 2 minutes and gently release. If it is too painful to firmly press this point, then rub or hold it for 30 seconds at a time.

## For wrist pain or strain:

## Acupressure Pericardium 6 (PC6): Inner Gate

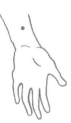

**Location:** in the center of the inner side of the forearm 3 finger widths above the wrist crease.
**Point Indications:** wrist pain, nausea, travel sickness, morning sickness.
**How to perform:** press and hold for 2 minutes and gently release. If it is too painful to firmly press this point, then rub or hold it for 30 seconds at a time.

## Acupressure Triple Warmer 5 (TW5): Outer Pass

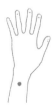

**Location:** three finger widths up from the outer wrist crease between two bones.
**Point indication:** injury to tendons, wrist pain.
**How to perform:** press and hold for 2 minutes and gently release. If it is too painful to firmly press this point, then rub or hold it for 30 seconds at a time.

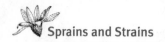

# Secondary Treatment

℞ **Homeopathic Rhus toxicodendron (Poison Ivy)**

**Quality:** general remedy for sprains and strains. The joint is hot and swollen. There is stiffness of the joint when it is first moved, and then after a while it limbers up and is better after continued motion.

**Mental-Emotional:** restlessness from pain, where the person constantly moves around.

**Better:** the injury is better from heat.

**Worse:** pain is worse in cold damp weather.

**Dose:** Rhus tox 30C (3 small pellets under tongue) every 4 hours up to 3 doses. Discontinue as symptoms improve.

**Follow-up:** Rhus tox 30C once a day until the sprain is healed.

*or*

℞ **Homeopathic Ruta graveolens (Rue Bitterwort)**

**Quality:** injuries to cartilage and tendons lying over a bone and around joints. Pulled tendons and ligaments, bruise to periosteum. The quality of pain is stiff and bruised.

**Worse:** the pain is worse in wet and cold weather.

**Dose:** Ruta 30C (3 small pellets under tongue) every 4 hours, up to 3 doses. Discontinue as symptoms improve.

*or*

℞ **Homeopathic Bryonia alba (Wild Hops)**

**General use and quality:** sprains and strains where the injured part is hot, red, and swollen. The pain is of a stitching, tearing quality.

**Generally:** the person may feel very thirsty.

**Mental-Emotional:** the person is irritable.

**Better:** the pain is better from rest and applying something cold.

**Worse:** the pain is worse with the slightest motion.

**Dose:** Bryonia 30C (3 small pellets under tongue) every 4 hours up to 3 doses. Discontinue as symptoms improve.

# Follow-up Treatment

### Homeopathic Ruta

Ruta 30C, once a day until the sprain is healed.

*or*

### Homeopathic Bryonia

Bryonia 30C, twice a day until the sprain is healed.

*or*

### Myoderm or Traumeel Homeopathic Creams

Topically as needed.

### Vitamin C (Ascorbic Acid)

**Form:** tablet, capsule, powder.
**Action:** promotes formation of collagen and elastin in skin, antioxidant, helps to prevent bruising.
**Indications:** bruising, burns and scalds, insect bites and stings, nosebleeds, poison ivy, scrapes, sprains and strains, sunburn.
**Dose:** 500 mg, 4 times a day with food for 2–4 weeks.
**Caution:** chewable vitamin C can damage tooth enamel and lead to cavity formation. Do not exceed 4,000 mg of vitamin C if pregnant. Do not combine with aspirin as stomach irritation or ulceration may occur.
**Note:** easy bruising may signal a deficiency in vitamin C.

### Bioflavanoids (rutin, hesperetin, hesperidin, quercetin)

**Form:** tablet, capsule (usually found together in a vitamin with vitamin C).
**Action:** reduces capillary fragility, antioxidant.

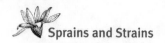 

**Indications:** bruising, burns and scalds, insect bites and stings, nosebleeds, poison ivy, scrapes, sprains and strains, sunburn.

**Dose:** 1000 mg per day.

**Caution:** very high doses may cause diarrhea.

# Stubbed Toe

## About Stubbed Toe

The fingers, toes, and tailbone are all areas of the body with lots of nerves. Because of the high concentration of nerves, crush injuries to toes are characterized often by shooting or sharp pains, and the pain may seem to radiate a distance to another part. There are two components to a crush injury: the bruising or bleeding under the skin from tiny blood vessels breaking and the nerve injury. The healing process involves reducing the inflammation so that the body re-absorbs the blood from the bruise, thus taking the pressure off the nerves and reducing the pain. It is important to rule out a fracture since the bones in toes are thin. A fracture would be suspected in any case of severe pain, extensive swelling, loss of normal function, or obvious deformity. Emergency medical treatment is then necessary.

**Minor:** bruising, pain, and slight swelling of toes.

**Serious:** the injury is serious when these symptoms or signs are present:

- excessive swelling
- cut or scrape around the joint
- loss of normal function (can't bend the toes)
- can't stand on the toes
- excessive pain that increases or doesn't go away in 2 days

**Caution:** when the injury is serious, seek medical attention.

## Primary Treatment

**Homeopathic Arnica montana (Leopard's Bane)**

> **Quality:** the part feels sore or bruised 'as if beaten'. Everything feels too hard.
> **Mental-Emotional:** mental shock after an injury or accident and the person may say there is nothing wrong even after a serious injury.
> **Dose:** Arnica 30C (3 small pellets under tongue) initially to reduce swelling. Discontinue homeopathic when symptoms improve.

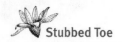

## Secondary Treatment

℞ **Homeopathic Hypericum (St. John's Wort)**

> **Quality:** injuries to nervous tissues. The pain is sharp and shooting.
> **Dose:** Hypericum 30C (3 small pellets under tongue) every 1–2 hours, up to 5 doses. Discontinue homeopathic when symptoms improve.

## Follow-up Treatment

℞ **Vitamin C (Ascorbic Acid)**

> **Form:** tablet, capsule, powder.
> **Action:** promotes formation of collagen and elastin in skin, antioxidant, helps to prevent bruising.
> **Indications:** bruising, burns and scalds, insect bites and stings, nosebleeds, poison ivy, scrapes, sprains and strains, sunburn.
> **Dose:** 500 mg, 4 times a day with food for 2–4 weeks.
> **Caution:** chewable vitamin C can damage tooth enamel and lead to cavity formation. Do not exceed 4,000 mg of vitamin C if pregnant. Do not combine with aspirin as stomach irritation or ulceration may occur.

℞ **Bioflavanoids (rutin, hesperetin, hesperidin, quercetin)**

> **Form:** tablet, capsule (usually found together in a vitamin with vitamin C).
> **Action:** reduces capillary fragility, antioxidant.
> **Indications:** bruising, burns and scalds, insect bites and stings, nosebleeds, poison ivy, scrapes, sprains and strains, sunburn.
> **Dose:** 1000 mg per day.
> **Caution:** very high doses may cause diarrhea.

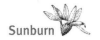

# Sunburn

## About Sunburns

A sunburn is caused by exposure to the sun's rays. Fair-skinned people are most susceptible to sunburns as their skin lacks the pigment melanin. Melanin is a substance which makes the skin appear darker and provides protection to the skin. The sun's ultraviolet rays are most powerful between 10 a.m. and 3 p.m. when the sun is highest in the sky.

Depending on the depth and severity of sunburned skin, burns are characterized as 1st, 2nd, and 3rd degree. First degree burns affect the surface layer. Second degree burns are deeper and cause released fluid creating blisters. Third degree burns are the most serious because they are the deepest. The nerves may be affected, causing a decreased pain sensation even though the burn may be severe.

One of the dangers of a sunburn is that a burn may not appear until a few hours to many hours after sun exposure. Cooling the skin immediately after a sunburn helps to prevent further damage.

| Type of Burn | Description | Type of Treatment |
|---|---|---|
| **1st degree burn** | • skin pink to red<br>• feels hot to touch<br>• dry<br>• slight swelling | Topical and Homeopathy |
| **2nd degree burn** | • red with blisters<br>• raw skin<br>• extreme pain | Homeopathy and seek medical attention.<br>Do not apply topical treatment. |
| **3rd degree burn** | • severe burn<br>• may have little or no pain<br>• pearly white to black skin | Seek emergency medical attention.<br>Do not apply topical treatment. |

**Caution:** Seek emergency medical treatment for any 2$^{nd}$ or 3$^{rd}$ degree sunburn that presents the following symptoms:

- swelling or blistering, especially where blisters open
- fever, nausea, chills
- burn interferes with breathing
- the person is under age 2 or over 50 years

Topical treatments should only be used for 1st degree burns where the skin is pink to red, there is tenderness or pain in the area, the wound is dry, and there is slight swelling. If the skin looks raw or blistered with clear fluid and extreme pain, this is a 2nd degree burn and only internal homeopathic medicines should be used. A 3rd degree burn may have pearly white to black skin and may be deep with no pain. No ointments should be used.

## Prevention

**Avoid Exposure**  Avoid prolonged exposure to the sun. Cover up with clothes and a hat. If you have fair skin, stay out of the sun during high UV times between 10 a.m. and 2 p.m.

**Sunscreen**  Use a sunscreen with SPF 15.

## Primary Treatment

**Cool Down**  Cool showers, baths, or compresses can be used to soothe the skin and prevent further worsening of the burn.

### For 1$^{st}$ Degree Burn *only*:

 **Homeopathic Urtica Ointment**

Apply Urtica urens (Stinging-nettle) ointment to sooth superficial burns, for red skin but no blistering. There may be a prickly, burning feeling.

*or*

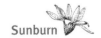

**Witch Hazel (Hamamelis virginiana)**

Apply a cold compress soaked in cold water and add 1–3 tsp of witch Hazel.

*or*

**Aloe vera**     Apply the gel from the inside of an aloe vera plant.

*or*

**Lavender Oil**     Apply 2–3 drops of lavender oil in 1 tsp of carrier oil such as almond oil.

*or*

**Myoderm Homeopathic Cream**

*or*

**Traumeel Homeopathic Cream**

**If the pain is not relieved by the ointment, or topical solution, take homeopathic Urtica urens or Cantharis internally:**

**Homeopathic Urtica urens (Stinging-nettle)**

**General quality:** for a first degree burn with red skin but no blistering. There may be a prickly, burning feeling.
**Dose:** Urtica urens 30C (3 small pellets under tongue) every 10 minutes or until the pain subsides, up to 5 doses. Discontinue homeopathic when symptoms improve.

*or*

**Homeopathic Cantharis (Spanish Fly)**

**General quality:** the quality of the pain is smarting, raw and burning. The burn is swollen. For the intense pain of burns and for second degree burns.
**Mental-Emotional:** the person may be angry or irritable with the pain.

**Better:** from cold application.
**Dose:** Cantharis 30C (3 small pellets under tongue) every 10 minutes or until the pain subsides, up to 5 doses. Discontinue homeopathic when symptoms improve.

*and*

**Vitamin E Oil**  Use vitamin E oil to help heal the burn after the pain has subsided or break open a vitamin E capsule and place the liquid on the burn twice a day.

## For 2<sup>nd</sup> Degree Burn:

### Homeopathic Cantharis (Spanish Fly)

**General quality:** the quality of the pain is smarting, raw and burning. The burn is swollen. For the intense pain of burns and for second degree burns.
**Mental-Emotional:** the person may be angry or irritable with the pain.
**Better:** from cold application.
**Dose:** Cantharis 30C (3 small pellets under tongue) every 10 minutes or until the pain subsides, up to 5 doses. Discontinue homeopathic when symptoms improve.

*or*

### Homeopathic Urtica urens (Stinging-nettle)

**General quality:** for a second degree burn with a stinging, prickly, burning feeling.
**Dose:** Urtica urens 30C (3 small pellets under tongue) every 10 minutes or until the pain subsides, up to 5 doses. Discontinue homeopathic when symptoms improve.

## For 3<sup>rd</sup> Degree Burn:

Get medical attention immediately.

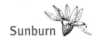

# Follow-up Treatment

**Vitamin A**   **Form:** capsule, tablet.
**Action:** growth and repair of new tissue, antioxidant, enhances immunity.
**Indications:** burns and scalds, poison plants, scrapes, sunburn.
**Dose:** 10,000 IU, 3 times a day for 2 weeks.
**Caution:** not to be taken over 10,000 IU if pregnant or you have liver disease. Vitamin A can be toxic if taken in large doses for extended periods.

**Vitamin C (Ascorbic Acid)**

**Form:** tablet, capsule, powder.
**Action:** promotes formation of collagen and elastin in skin, antioxidant, helps to prevent bruising.
**Indications:** bruising, burns and scalds, insect bites and stings, nosebleeds, poison ivy, scrapes, sprains and strains, sunburn.
**Dose:** 500 mg, 4 times a day with food for 2–4 weeks.
**Caution:** chewable vitamin C can damage tooth enamel and lead to cavity formation. Do not exceed 4,000 mg of vitamin C if pregnant. Do not combine with aspirin as stomach irritation or ulceration may occur.

**Vitamin E**   **Form:** internally, capsules; topically, break open a capsule or apply oil from a container.
**Action:** antioxidant, facilitates tissue repair, reduces scarring, strengthens capillaries.
**Indications:** burns and scalds, scrapes, sunburn
**Dose:** 400 IU internally. Topically apply a thin layer of oil to affected area.
**Caution:** internally, vitamin E in large doses can elevate blood pressure. Do not take large doses of vitamin E (over 1000 IU) if on blood thinners.
**Contraindication:** externally, do not use immediately on 2nd or 3rd degree burns until the top layer of skin is healing over.

**Ⓡ Mineral Zinc**   **Form:** tablet, capsule.
**Action:** antioxidant, repair of tissue especially for collagen formation in skin and protein synthesis.
**Indications:** burns and scalds, poison ivy, scrapes, sunburn.
**Dose:** 30 mg per day for 2–4 weeks.
**Caution:** zinc supplements can cause nausea if taken in doses higher than 30 mg at one time. Do not take more than 100 mg of zinc per day.
**Note:** poor wound healing is one sign of deficiency of zinc.

**Ⓡ Bioflavanoids (rutin, hesperetin, hesperidin, quercetin)**

**Form:** tablet, capsule (usually found together in a vitamin with vitamin C).
**Action:** reduces capillary fragility, antioxidant.
**Indications:** bruising, burns and scalds, insect bites and stings, nosebleeds, poison ivy, scrapes, sprains and strains, sunburn.
**Dose:** 1000 mg per day.
**Caution:** very high doses may cause diarrhea.

**Ⓡ Essential Fatty Acids
(from black currant oil, flax seed oil, evening primrose oil)**

**Form:** capsules.
**Action:** needed for repair of cells.
**Indications:** burns and scalds, poison ivy, scrapes, sunburn.
**Dose:** 1000 mg, 3 times a day with food.
**Caution:** consult your naturopathic doctor before taking if you are on anti-clotting medication (blood thinners).
**Note:** a deficiency of essential fatty acids may be a cause of poor wound healing.

# Tailbone Injury

## About Tailbone Injury

The fingers, toes, and tailbone are all areas of the body with lots of nerves. Because of the high concentration of nerves, crush injuries to the tailbone are characterized often by shooting or sharp pains and the pain may seem to radiate a distance to another part. There are two components to a crush injury: the bruising or bleeding under the skin from tiny blood vessels breaking and the nerve injury. The healing process involves reducing the inflammation so that the body re-absorbs the blood from the bruise, thus taking the pressure off the nerves and reducing the pain. It is important to rule out a fracture since the bones in the tailbone are thin. A fracture would be suspected in any case of severe pain, extensive swelling, loss of normal function, or obvious deformity. Emergency medical treatment is then necessary.

**Minor:** slight swelling and pain.

**Serious:** increased pain, lots of swelling, where it is impossible to sit down because of the pain.

**Caution:** if pain persists, seek medical attention to determine if there is a fracture.

## Primary Treatment

**Homeopathic Arnica montana (Leopard's Bane)**

> **Quality:** the part feels sore or bruised 'as if beaten'. Everything feels too hard.
> **Mental-Emotional:** mental shock after an injury or accident and the person may say there is nothing wrong even after a serious injury.
> **Dose:** Arnica 30C (3 small pellets under tongue) initially to reduce inflammation.

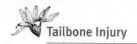 

## Secondary Treatment

℞ **Homeopathic Hypericum (St. John's Wort)**

> **General use and quality:** injuries to nervous tissues where the pain is sharp and shooting.
> **Dose:** Hypericum 30C (3 small pellets under tongue) every 1–2 hours, up to 5 doses. Discontinue homeopathic when symptoms improve.

## Follow-up Treatment

℞ **Vitamin C (Ascorbic Acid)**

> **Form:** tablet, capsule, powder.
> **Action:** promotes formation of collagen and elastin in skin, antioxidant, helps to prevent bruising.
> **Indications:** bruising, burns and scalds, insect bites and stings, nosebleeds, poison ivy, scrapes, sprains and strains, sunburn.
> **Dose:** 500 mg, 4 times a day with food for 2–4 weeks.
> **Caution:** chewable vitamin C can damage tooth enamel and lead to cavity formation. Do not exceed 4,000 mg of vitamin C if pregnant. Do not combine with aspirin as stomach irritation or ulceration may occur.

℞ **Bioflavanoids (rutin, hesperetin, hesperidin, quercetin)**

> **Form:** tablet, capsule (usually found together in a vitamin with vitamin C).
> **Action:** reduces capillary fragility, antioxidant.
> **Indications:** bruising, burns and scalds, insect bites and stings, nosebleeds, poison ivy, scrapes, sprains and strains, sunburn.
> **Dose:** 1000 mg per day.
> **Caution:** very high doses may cause diarrhea.

# Travel Conditions

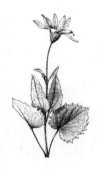

# Travel Conditions

When traveling, especially with children, there are several minor conditions which may respond to natural medicines. By assembling a first aid kit specifically for the car, train, bus, or plane, you can prevent or relieve many of these conditions.

For conditions of constipation and diarrhea also see the discussion and treatments in the Minor Conditions section.

*Special Note:* when taking homeopathic medicines on an airplane, it is best to avoid having them x-rayed as this may affect their potency.

# Diarrhea & Constipation

## About Diarrhea and Constipation while Traveling

Most traveler's diarrhea is due primarily to contamination of drinking water and secondarily to contamination of food. Children are most susceptible as well as those with low stomach acid and immunity. Traveler's constipation is due to irregular meals, lack of exercise, dehydration, and eating too many refined, processed foods that are low in fiber.

## Prevention

**Purify Water**   To prevent traveler's diarrhea, such as cholera, several precautions should be taken, including boiling water to be used for drinking and for tooth brushing, and avoiding uncooked vegetables or undercooked fish or shellfish.

**Drink Water**   Do not avoid drinking water, however, or the result may be constipation. Drink 6 – 8 glasses of purified or bottled water daily while traveling, especially while traveling in airplanes.

**Eat as the Natives Do**

When dining in a foreign country, it is important to eat as the natives do. Often food is highly spiced with cayenne pepper (Capsicum frutescens) and garlic (Allium sativum). Cayenne pepper is antibacterial and a gastric stimulant which helps to kill the bacteria that may be in the food or water. Garlic has antibacterial and antiparasitic action. Choose high fiber foods such as beans, cooked vegetables, and whole grains. Eat regular meals.

℞ **Citricidal™ Liquid Concentrate (Professional Brand)**

> **Form:** liquid concentrate.
> **Action:** antibacterial, antifungal.
> **Dose:** 3–5 drops in 5–6 oz of water, in morning to prevent traveler's diarrhea, 2–3 times daily to treat diarrhea.
> **Caution:** avoid contact with eyes. Do not use undiluted.
> **Note:** available from a naturopathic doctor or health care professional.

*or*

℞ **Nutribiotic™ Liquid Grapefruit Seed Extract**

> **Form:** liquid concentrate.
> **Action:** antibacterial, antifungal.
> **Dose:** 5–15 drops in 5–6 oz of water, in morning to prevent traveler's diarrhea, 2–3 times daily to treat diarrhea.
> **Caution:** avoid contact with eyes. Do not use undiluted.
> **Note:** available from health food stores.

## Treatment

Travel with a complete 'Traveler's First Aid Kit' for preparing Re-hydrating liquids.

℞ **World Health Organization Formula for Diarrhea**

> 3.5 g sodium chloride (salt)
> 2.5 g sodium bicarbonate (baking soda)
> 1.5 g potassium chloride
> 20 g glucose
> 1 liter purified water

> See other treatments for Diarrhea and Constipation in 'Minor Conditions' section.

# Earache

## About Earache while Traveling

An earache can be caused by an infection in the ear, but an earache on a plane can occur if the eustachian tube is blocked. The eustachian tube runs between the ear and the throat behind the jawbone. This tube allows for the pressure to equalize in the ear and can be blocked if your nose is stuffed up or you have a cold.

When an airplane is ascending or descending, changes in air pressure occur. This pressure can feel like a stuffiness or sharp pain in the eardrum. When the pressure is equal between the inner ear and the outside, the pain and discomfort is relieved. Swallowing, yawning, or moving the jaw helps to relieve the build-up of pressure.

## Primary Treatment

### Unblock the Eustachian Tube

Swallow saliva, suck on a candy, or chew gum upon take off and landing, move your jaw around to allow the pressure to become equal.

### Acupressure Triple Warmer 17 (TW17): Wind Screen

**Location:** behind the earlobe.
**Point indication:** relieves toothache and ear pain.
**How to perform:** press gently and make circular motions to stimulate this point with your fingers.

### Acupressure Small Intestine 19 (SI19): Listening Place

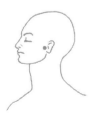

**Location:** in front of the opening to the ear. When the jaw is moved up and down, an indentation can be felt.
**Point indication:** relieves pressure inside the ear, earaches, toothaches.
**How to perform:** Press gently and make small circles to stimulate this point with the mouth open

# Secondary Treatment

℞ **Homeopathic Pulsatilla (Windflower)**

> **Quality:** acute earaches, earaches in airplanes.
> **General:** no thirst.
> **Mental-Emotional:** tearfulness, moodiness, wants attention.
> **Better:** in open air.
> **Worse:** in a stuffy airplane.
> **Dose:** Pulsatilla 30C (3 small pellets under tongue) every 15 minutes or until pain subsides up to 3 doses.

*or*

℞ **Homeopathic Kalium muraticum (Potassium Chloride)**

> **General use and quality:** eustachian tube and middle ear infections, fluid in the ear, plugged ear, nose and throat infections with a stringy discharge.
> **Better:** from cold drinks, from rubbing the area.
> **Worse:** in fresh air, in damp weather.
> **Note:** use Kali muraticum 6X or 12X (3 small pellets under tongue) one dose the day before the airplane ride. Take one dose the same day of the airplane ride at least a few hours before. Take one dose up to every 15 minutes if needed on the airplane ride.

# Fear of Flying

## About Fear of Flying while Traveling

This is a condition which involves nervousness or anxiety and may be related to a feeling of not being in control.

**Minor:** restlessness, anxiety, nervousness, heart pounding, rapid breathing, sweaty palms. Symptoms do not last more than one day.

**Serious:** signs of shock which may include paleness with sweating, cold limbs, rapid weak pulse, person feels cold and clammy to touch, person feels weak and faint. Prolonged feelings of anxiety and nervousness.

**Caution:** Alert a flight attendant if someone is showing signs of shock. If anxiety and nervousness last more than a few days, seek medical attention.

## Primary Treatment

**Relaxation Exercises**

Relaxation exercises, such as deep breathing; positive self talk, such as 'I am calm and peaceful'.

**Acupressure Heart 7 (HE7): Spirit Gate**

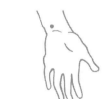

**Location:** on the wrist crease on the inner side of the tendon closest to the little finger.
**Point action and indication:** relieves anxiety, nervousness, fear.
**How to perform:** breathe deeply as you press firmly and hold for two minutes. You may feel a more sharp or radiating feeling at this point.

**Acupressure Conception Vessel 17 (CV17): Sea of Tranquility**

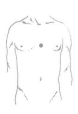

**Location:** three finger widths up from the joining of the rib cage on the breastbone in the midline of the body.
**Point action and indication:** relieves anxiety, nervousness, sensation of fullness in the chest. Helps deep breathing.

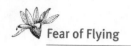 

**How to perform:** measure three finger widths up from base of joining of rib cage. Press firmly and hold, taking deep breaths for two minutes.

℞ **Bach Flower Rescue Remedy**

**Indication/emotion:** nervousness, trembling, anxiety, fear, panic, apprehension.

## Secondary Treatment

℞ Homeopathic Aconitum napellus (Monkshood)

**Mental-Emotional:** fear of flying with great anxiety and restlessness.
**Worse:** after exposure to cold dry wind.
**Dose:** Aconite 30C (3 small pellets under tongue) every 15 minutes or until symptoms improve, up to 3 doses.

*or*

℞ Homeopathic Argentum Nitricum (Nitrate of Silver)

**Quality:** fear of flying with trembling, and impulsive thoughts.
**Mental-Emotional:** fear of heights and claustrophobia, nervousness.
**Better:** fresh air.
**Worse:** warmth.
**Dose:** Arg Nit 30C (3 small pellets under tongue) every 15 minutes or until symptoms improve, up to 3 doses.

*or*

℞ Homeopathic Arsenicum album (Arsenic Acid)

**General use and quality:** fear of flying with restlessness and fear of death, generally fearful and restless.
**General Symptoms:** burning pains.
**Mental-Emotional:** anxiety, nervousness, fear of death.
**Better:** Heat, warmth.
**Worse:** Cold, being alone.
**Dose:** Arsenicum 30C (3 small pellets under tongue) every 15 minutes or until symptoms improve, up to 3 doses.

# Homesickness

## About Homesickness while Traveling

This is a feeling of longing for being back home, often experienced by children when going to an unfamiliar setting such as to camp. As a person gets used to a new surrounding, homesickness may subside. Certain people find it easier to adapt to new surroundings than others.

**Minor:** feeling sad and wanting to return home.

**Serious:** if homesickness lasts for more than a few days, seek medical attention.

## Primary Treatment

**Bach Flower Remedy Honeysuckle**

> **Indication/emotion:** homesickness, living in the past.
> **Dose:** 1 dropper full of diluted tincture (2 oz water and 3 drops tincture), 3–4 times a day or more often if the feeling of homesickness persists.

# Jet Lag

## About Jet Lag while Traveling

This is a condition that happens when a person travels through one or more time zones in a short period of time, usually via airplane. Symptoms vary from person to person and may include tiredness, weakness, trembling, fatigue, dizziness, drowsiness, or insomnia, which occur 1–2 days after travel until the body adjusts to the change in day and night. Symptoms worsen the more time zones crossed. Jet lag is generally worse going from west to east. The body's light-dark clock is regulated by the pineal gland. This light-sensitive gland must adjust to new daylight cycles, and this process can take from a few days to two weeks to occur.

**Minor:** tiredness, weakness, trembling, fatigue, and dizziness.

**Serious:** if symptoms are related to loss of fluid or not having enough fluids, it may indicate dehydration (see heat exhaustion) if symptoms persist more than 3 days.

## Primary Treatment

Ⓡ **Homeopathic Arnica montana (Leopard's Bane)**

> **Mental-Emotional:** mental shock and exhaustion of jet lag.
> **Dose:** Arnica 30C (3 small pellets under tongue) twice a day for the first day. Discontinue once symptoms improve.

*or*

Ⓡ **Homeopathic Cocculus (Indian Cockle)**

> **Quality:** the person has nausea, is weak, trembling, with a numb empty feeling.
> **Mental-Emotional:** Mentally slow and lack of sleep makes time seem to pass by too fast.
> **Better:** lying and must lie down.
> **Worse:** from sitting, loss of sleep, or the smell of food.
> **Dose:** Cocculus 30C (3 small pellets under tongue) twice a day for the first day. Discontinue once symptoms improve.

*or*

## Homeopathic Gelsemium (Yellow Jasmine)

**General use and quality:** jet lag with trembling, fatigue and weakness, dullness, dizziness, drowsiness. There may be diarrhea.

**Mental-Emotional:** anticipatory nervousness.

**Dose:** Gelsemium 30C (3 small pellets under tongue) twice a day for the first day. Discontinue once symptoms improve.

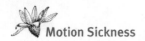 

# Motion Sickness

## About Motion Sickness while Traveling

Motion sickness is a feeling of disorientation and nausea, possibly with vomiting, that results from an upset in the balance mechanisms of the ear. There are three tubes that make-up the balance mechanism in the ear which are placed in different planes. The tubes have small sensitive hairs inside them which respond to the flow of fluid and tell us which way we are standing. When you are moving in one or even two directions at once, the body is able to cope, but when the balance mechanisms detect that you are moving in all three directions at once, motion sickness can occur.

Motion sickness may be a result of an adaptive evolutionary mechanism. If your balance mechanisms were going in all three directions at once, you were probably in the jaws of a hungry predator and were likely to be lunch. Vomiting may have been an adaptive way to be less appetizing to a predator. Because the body can cope with movement in two directions, but not three, it is important to stare at the horizon, or sit in the front seat of a car to keep the head still in one direction. Motion sickness usually resolves once you stop moving.

**Minor:** nausea, the feeling that you are going to throw up.

**Serious:** prolonged vomiting and signs of dehydration such as:

- sunken eyes
- pale
- dizziness when standing up
- sleepiness
- dry mouth
- weakness
- confusion
- intense thirst

# Prevention

## Maintain Equilibrium

Sit in the front seat of the automobile. Try to look out the front window or at the horizon. Open a window. Avoid reading while in motion.

## Primary Treatment

### Acupressure Pericardium 6 (PC6): Inner Gate

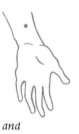

**Point indications:** nausea, travel sickness, morning sickness.
**Point location:** in the center of the inner side of the forearm, 3 finger widths above the wrist crease.
**How to perform:** apply firm pressure for 2 minutes then gently let go. Repeat whenever you feel nausea.

*and*

### Acupressure Liver 3 (LV3): Bigger Rushing

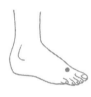

**Point indications:** nausea.
**Point location:** in the webbing on top of the foot between the big toe and the second toe, 2 finger widths above the crease of these 2 toes.
**How to perform:** Locate the point by placing index and middle fingers together to measure from the crease of the web of the toes up 2 finger widths to the point. Use your index finger to press firmly enough to cause tenderness to your tolerance. Hold for 1 minute, then repeat with other foot. Repeat when you feel nausea.

*and/or*

### Crystallized Ginger (Zingiber officinalis)

**Actions:** prevents vomiting.
**Dose:** crystallized ginger 1 inch-square piece chewed just before and during the journey, up to 5 pieces per hour.

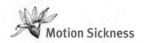 

**Caution:** avoid excessive amounts of ginger in stomach ulcers, inflammation of the digestive tract or in early pregnancy.

*and/or*

### Peppermint: Mentha piperita

**Actions:** antispasmodic, prevents vomiting.
**Dose:** 10–60 drops of tincture taken in a half a glass of water during the car trip. Drink as often as needed up to 180 drops in 3 hours. Or 1 teaspoonful in 1 cup of water. Pour boiling water over leaves and let steep for 10 minutes. Take as often as necessary.
**Caution:** do not give to children or babies. Do not use if breast feeding as too much can reduce milk flow. Contraindications: do not use if you have a hiatal hernia.

*or*

### Homeopathic Cocculus (Indian Cockle)

**Quality:** dizziness where everything around the person is spinning. The person has nausea, is weak, trembling, with a numb empty feeling.
**Mental-Emotional:** mentally slow and lack of sleep makes time seem to pass by too fast.
**Better:** lying and must lie down.
**Worse:** from sitting, loss of sleep, or the smell of food.
**Dose:** Cocculus 30C (3 small pellets under tongue) 2 days prior to the trip if you are prone to travel sickness, or during the trip every half hour for up to 5 doses. Discontinue homeopathic when symptoms improve.

*or*

### Homeopathic Nux vomica (Poison Nut)

**Quality:** motion sickness with queasiness, chills, and there may be a headache at the back of the head or over one eye. There may also be constipation from traveling.

**General:** person feels chilly, is very sensitive to light, noise, odors.
**Mental-Emotional:** irritable and oversensitive.
**Worse:** from food, tobacco smoke and coffee.
**Dose:** Nux vomica 30C (3 small pellets under tongue) every half hour for up to 5 doses. Discontinue homeopathic when symptoms improve.

*or*

## Homeopathic Tabaccum (Tobacco)

**Quality:** motion sickness with nausea, dizziness and faintness, chills, sweating, sensation of a band around the head.
**General Symptoms:** person may be pale and icy cold.
**Mental-Emotional:** disconnected.
**Worse:** near tobacco smoke.
**Dose:** Tabacum 30C (3 small pellets under tongue) every half hour for up to 5 doses. Discontinue homeopathic when symptoms improve.

# 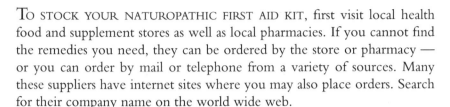 *Naturopathic Medicine Suppliers Directory*

To STOCK YOUR NATUROPATHIC FIRST AID KIT, first visit local health food and supplement stores as well as local pharmacies. If you cannot find the remedies you need, they can be ordered by the store or pharmacy — or you can order by mail or telephone from a variety of sources. Many these suppliers have internet sites where you may also place orders. Search for their company name on the world wide web.

## Canadian Sources for Botanical & Herbal Remedies

**Christmas Natural Foods**
Unit 201, 8173 108th St
Surrey, BC V3W 4G1

**Ferlow Brothers Ltd.**
PO Box 3197
Mission, BC V2V 4J4
(604) 820-1777

**Herbal Solutions**
14931 Thift Ave
White Rock, BC V4B 2J8
(604) 535-5222

**Global Botanicals**
545 Welham Rd
Barrie, ON L4N 8Z7
(800) 887-6009

**St Francis Herb Farm Inc**
PO Box 29
Combermere, ON K0J 1L0
(800) 219-6226

## Canadian Sources for Homeopathic Medicines

**Boiron Canada Inc.**
816 Guimond St
Longueuil, QC J4G 1T5
(800) 361-1010

**Dolisos**
1400 Hocquart
Saint Bruno, QC J3V 6E1
Tel. 1-800-461-1400

**Dolisos Homeopathics**
PO Box 56603
861 Warden Ave
Markham, ON L3R 0M6

**Dr Reckeweg**
**Homeopathic Specialties**
518 Meloche Ave
Dorval, QC H9P 2T2
(514) 631-6627
(800) 361-6663

**Homéocan Inc.**
1900 St. Catherine Street East
Montréal, QC H2K 1H5

**Seroyal Canada**
44 East Beaver Creek Rd, Suite 17
Richmond Hill, ON L4B 1G8
(800) 263-5861

Thompson's Homeopathic Supplies
844 Yonge Street
Toronto, ON M4W 2H1

# American Sources for Botanical & Herbal Remedies

**Dances with Herbs**
PO Box 1100
Idyllwild, CA 92549
(775) 766-0219

**McZand Herbal Inc.**
PO Box 5312
Santa Monica, CA 90409
(310) 822-0500

**Herbs, Etc.**
1341 Rufina Circle
Santa Fe, NM 87501
(800) 634-3727

**Nature's Herbs**
PO Box 336
Orem, UT 84059
(800) HERBALS

**Herb-Pharm**
PO Box 116,
William, OR 97544
(503) 846-6262

# American Sources for Homeopathic Medicines

**B and T**
281 Circadian Way,
Santa Rosa, CA 95407

**BHI**
11600 Cochiti SE
Albuquerque, NM 87123

**Bioforce of America, Ltd.**
PO Box 507
Kinderhook, NY 12106

**Boericke and Tafel, Inc.**
1011 Arch Street
Philadelphia, PA 19107
(215) 922-2967

**Boiron**
6 Campus Boulevard,
Building A
Newton Square, PA 19073

**Boiron-Borneman**
1208 Amosland Road
Norwood, PA 19074
(215) 532-2035

**Dolisos America, Inc.**
3014 Rigel Ave
Las Vegas, NV 89102
(702) 871-7153

**Hahnemann Pharmacy**
828 San Pablo Ave
Albany, CA 94706
(510) 527-3003

**HoboN**
4594 Enterprise Ave
Naples, FL 33942

**Homeopathic Educational Services**
2124 Kittredge St
Berkeley, CA 94704
(510) 649-8930

**Humphreys**
63 Meadow Rd
Rutherford, NJ 07070

**Luyties**
P.O. Box 8080
St. Louis, MO 63165-8080

**Luyties Pharmaceutical Company**
4200 Laclede Ave
St. Louis, MO 63108
(800) 325-8080

**NF Formulas Inc.**
9775 SW Commerce Circle, C-5
Wilsonville, OR 97070-9602
(800)547-4891

**Nature's Way Products**
10 Mountain Springs Parkway
Springville, UT 84663
(800) 489-1520

**Similisan Corp.**
1321D South Central Ave
Kent, WA 98003

**Standard Homeopathic Co.**
210 West 131 St
Los Angeles, CA 90061

**Standard Homeopathic Company**
PO Box 61604
436 West Eighth St
Los Angeles, CA 90014
(213) 321-4284

**Super Salve**
606 Lake Mary Rd
Flagstaff, AZ 86001
(602) 774-8910

**Waleda**
841 South Main St
Spring Valley, NY 10977

**Washington Homepathic Products**
4914 Del Ray Ave
Bethesada, MD 20814

**Wyoming Wildcrafters**
Wilson, WY 80304
(307) 733-6731

## Sources for Bach Flower Remedies

**Nelson Bach**
PO Box 62554
Cedar Hills R.P.O.
Surrey, BC V3V 7V6

**Ellon Bach USA, Inc.**
644 Merrick Rd
Lynbrook, NY 11563
(516) 593-2206

**Homeopathic Educational Services**
2124 Kittredge St
Berkeley, CA 94704
(510)649-0294

## Sources for Specialty Creams & Gels

**'Traumeel
Homeopathic Cream'**
Manufactured by Heel
Distributed by Acti-Form Ltd.
(888) 379-4335

**'Apis Homeopathic Gel'**
Doliso
1400 Hocquart
Saint Bruno, QC J3V 6E1
(800) 461-1400

**'Myoderm
Homeopathic Cream'**
NF Formulas Inc.
9775 SW Commerce Circle, C-5
Wilsonville, OR 97070-9602
(800) 547-4891

**'Solar Cream'**
Derma Med Pharmaceuticals Inc.
1103-13351 Commerce Parkway
Richmond, BC V6V 2X7
(604) 273-6101

## Sources for Insect Repellants

**All Terrain Company**
'All Terrain Herbal Armor'
3275 Corporate Views
Vista, CA 92083
(800) 2INSECT

**Aubrey Organics**
'Gone'
4419 North Manhattan Ave
Tampa, FL 33614
(800) 282-7379

**IMHOTP**
Outdoor Herbal Spray
'The Bug Disenchanter'
PO Box 183
Ruby, NY 12475
(800) 677-8577

**Penn Herb Co.**
'Buzz Away'
10601 Decatur Rd
Philadelphia, PA 19154
(800) 523-9971
www.pennherb.com

**St Francis Herb Farm Inc**
'Ledum Away'
PO Box 29
Combermere, ON K0J 1L0
(800) 219-6226

## Sources for Traveler's Diarrhea Remedies

**Ecotrend Products Ltd**
Nutribiotic™ Liquid Grapefruit
Seed Extract
188 W 6th Ave, FL 202
Vancouver, BC V5Y 1K6
(800) 665-7065

**Citricidal Liquid Concentrate**
(Professional Brand)

Available from your naturopathic
doctor or other health care
professional.

# ✳ *Naturopathic References and Resources* ✳

IN RESEARCHING AND WRITING *Naturopathic First Aid*, a number of articles and books were consulted. The reader interested in learning more about naturopathic first aid and naturopathic medicine in general may find this list of references valuable.

Ali, Dr E., Grant, Dr G., Nakla, Dr S. 1999. The tea tree oil bible. Toronto, ON: Ages Publications.

Aikins, M.P. 1998. Alternative therapies for nausea and vomiting of pregnancy. Obstetrics and Gynecology, 91(1):149-55.

Balch, J.F., Balch, P.A. 1997. Prescription for nutritional healing. Garden City, NY: Avery Publishing Group.

Berkow, R., Fletcher, A.J. et al. 1992. The Merck manual of diagnosis and therapy. Rathway, NJ: Merck and Co Inc.

Boericke, W. M.D. 1927. Pocket manual of homeopathic materia medica. Santa Rosa, CA: Boericke and Tafel Inc.

Britton, J., Kircher, R. 1998. The complete book of home herbal remedies. Willowdale, ON: Firefly Books Ltd.

Buchbauer G., Jirovetz, L. et al., 1991. Aromatherapy: Evidence for sedative effects of the essential oil of lavender after inhalation. Z Naturforsch [C], Nov-Dec;46(11-12):1067-72.

Dowling R.J. et al. 1985. Use of fat emulsions, in M Deitel, Ed. Nutrition in Clinical Surgery. Baltimore, Williams and Wilkins: 139-47.

Ellis, A., Wiseman, N., Boss, K. 1991. Fundamentals of Chinese acupuncture. Brookline, MA: Paradigm Publications.

Fulghum D.D. 1977. Ascorbic acid revisited. Arch Dermatol, 113(1):91-92.

Gach, M.R. 1990. Acupressure's potent points: A guide to self-care for common ailments. Toronto, ON: Bantam Books.

Gerber, L.E., Erdman, J.W. Jr. 1981. Wound healing in rats fed small supplements of retinyl acetate, beta-carotene or retinoic acid. Fed Proc, Mar 2;3453:838.

Goldstein R. et al. 1990. Effect of vitamin E and allopurinol on lipid peroxide and glutathione levels in acute skin grafts. J. Invest Dermatol, 95:470.

Hammond, C. 1995. The complete family guide to homeopathy: An illustrated encyclopedia of safe and effective remedies. Toronto, ON: Penguin Books Ltd.

Heinerman, J. 1993. First aid with herbs: tried and true health care in emergencies and minor illnesses. New Canaan, CT: Keats Publishing Inc.

Hoffmann, D. 1992. Therapeutic herbalism. Santa Rosa, CA: David Hoffmann Inc.

Jacobs, J. 1996. The encyclopedia of alternative medicine. Toronto, ON: Stoddart Publishing Company Ltd.

Jonas, W.B., Jacobs, J. 1996. Healing with homeopathy: The complete guide. New York, NY: Warner Books.

Kim, J.E., Shklar, G. 1983. The effect of vitamin E on the healing of gingival wounds in rats. J. Peridontol, 54:305.

Lis-Balchin, M., Hart, S. 1997. A preliminary study of the affect of essential oils on skeletal and smooth muscle in vitro. Journal of Ethnopharmacology Nov;58(3):183-7.

Lockie, A., Geddes, N. 1995. The complete guide to homeopathy: the principles and practice of treatment. Westmount, QC: The Readers Digest Association of Canada Ltd.

Lust, J., Tierra, M. 1990. The natural remedy bible. Toronto ON: Pocket Books.

Martin, A. 1996. The use of antioxidants in healing. Dermatology and Surgery, Feb; 22(2):156-60.

Morrison, R. 1993. Desktop guide to keynotes and confirmatory symptoms. Albany, CA: Hahnemann Clinic Publishing.

Murad S. et al. 1981. Regulation of collagen synthesis by ascorbic acid. Proc Natl Acad Sci USA,78(5):2879-82.

Murat, Dr B., Stewart, Dr G. Do I need to see the doctor? A guide for treating common minor ailments at home. Huntsville, ON: Doc'N A Book Publishing.

Nenoff, P., Haustein, U.F., Brandt, W. 1996. Antifungal activity of the essential oil of Melaleuca alternifolia (tea tree oil) against pathogenic fungi in vitro. Skin Pharmacology 9(6): 388-94.

Ody, P. 1993. The complete medicinal herbal. Toronto, ON: Key Porter Books.

Ringsdorf, W.M. Jr, Cheraskin, E. 1982. Vitamin C and human wound healing. Oral Surg 53(3):231-36.

Schroyens, F. 1995. Synthesis: repertorium homeopathicum syntheticum. London, UK: Homeopathic Book Publishers.

Sieradzki, E., Olejarz, E. et al. 1998. The effect of selenium and vitamin E on the healing process of experimental corneal lesions in the eye of the rabbit. Klin Oczna 100(2):85-8.

Sherman, J.A. 1993. The complete botanical prescriber. Sand, OR: NF Publishers.

Shealy, C. 1996. The complete family guide to alternative medicine: an illustrated encyclopedia of natural healing.

Tisserand, R., Balacs, T. 1995. Essential oil safety: A guide for health care professionals. New York, NY: Churchill Livingstone.

Thompson, D. 1999. Mosquito, mosquito go away. Townsend Letter for Doctors and Patients, 190.

Ullman, J.R. 2000. Homeopathic outdoor kit. Townsend Letter for Doctors and Patients, July;204:49-50.

Valentine, G., Haliburton, B. 1995. First on the scene: The complete guide to first aid and CPR. Ottawa, ON: St. John Ambulance.

Werbach, M.R. 1996. Nutritional influences on illness: A sourcebook of clinical research. Tarzana, CA: Third Line Press.

Williams, R.M. 2000. Health risks and environmental issues: DEET Alert!" Townsend Letter for Doctors and Patients, July;204:38-39.

Zand, J., Walton, R., Roundtree, B. 1994. Smart Medicine for a healthier child. Garden City, NY: Avery Publishing Group.

Zydlo, S.M., Hill, J.A. 1990. The American Medical Association Handbook of First Aid and Emergency Care. New York, NY: Random House.